OCCUPATIONAL
LOW BACK
PAIN

Aggressive Nonsurgical Care

OCCUPATIONAL LOW BACK PAIN

Aggressive Nonsurgical Care

Edited by

Bryan D. Kaplansky, M.D.

CRC Press

Boca Raton   London   New York   Washington, D.C.

Library of Congress Cataloging-in-Publication Data

Catalog record is available from the Library of Congress.

Overview

Occupational low back pain remains the most common musculoskeletal condition affecting the working population, representing 25 to 40% of Worker's Compensation claims. The cost of occupational low back pain in the United States has been estimated to be up to $100 billion dollars per year.[1] The enormous socioeconomic cost of occupational low back pain and disability has forced health care providers and industry personnel to focus on cost-effective and efficacious strategies for diagnostic testing, treatment, and prevention of low back pain disorders. This emphasis towards cost-effective and scientifically proven treatment has been driven by the scrutiny associated with changes in the economic climate of health care. The evolving process of caring for the worker with low back pain is further complicated by the quagmire of the various opinions of health care providers concerning what is appropriate and proper care for the injured worker. Numerous providers care for individuals with low back disorders with varying treatment outcomes. As the science of spine care evolves, it has become readily apparent that a broad background in musculoskeletal medicine is necessary in delivering appropriate care for workers with low back pain. A multidisciplinary approach to occupational low back pain is considered the most effective strategy.

This textbook initially covers the diagnostic approach to occupational low back pain. The history and physical examination, and the appropriate utilization of imaging studies and electrodiagnostic studies, as well as the appropriate utilization of diagnostic spinal injections are covered. Also the use of functional capacity evaluations is reviewed. In the treatment section, the aspects of exercise, pharmacologic treatment, therapeutic injection treatment, manual medicine, modalities, and orthotics are covered. This textbook also covers the surgical indications for low back disorders. Finally, the last chapter covers the important topic of low back pain prevention. Chronic low back pain programs and the evaluation and treatment of associated psychological disorders are not covered here. The emphasis of this textbook is the aggressive nonsurgical approach to occupational low back pain. Primarily written by nonsurgeons, each expert has covered the appropriate steps that can be undertaken addressing this important topic involving the workplace.

Reference

1. Frymoyer, J. W. Cost and control of industrial musculoskeletal injuries, in *Musculoskeletal Disorders in the Workplace: Principles and Practice*, Nordin, M., Andersson, G., and Pope, M., eds., Chicago: Mosby, 1997, 62–71.

Contributors

Mayra I. Alfonso, M.D.
Postdoctoral Research Fellow
Department of Physical Medicine
and Rehabilitation
Medical College of Wisconsin
Milwaukee, WI

James W. Atchison, D.O.
Associate Professor and Chief
Division of Physical Medicine
and Rehabilitation
Department of Orthopaedics
and Rehabilitation
University of Florida
College of Medicine
Gainesville, FL

Andrew J. Haig, M.D.
Assistant Professor
Department of Physical Medicine
and Rehabilitation
Medical Director
The Spine Program / University of
Michigan Health System
Ann Arbor, MI

Barbara A. Heller, D.O., R.P.T.
Chicago, IL

Bryan D. Kaplansky, M.D.
Orthopaedics Northeast, P.C.
Fort Wayne, IN

Myron M. LaBan, M.D.,
FACP, MMSc, LMT, PC
Director Physical Medicine and
Rehabilitation
William Beaumont Hospital
Royal Oak, MI

Howard I. Levy, M.D.
Assistant Professor of Physical
Medicine and Rehabilitation
Assistant Professor of Orthopaedics
EmoryUniversity
School of Medicine
Atlanta, GA

Gerard A. Malanga, M.D.
Director Sports, Spine and
Orthopedic Rehabilitation
Kessler Institute for Rehabilitation
West Orange, NJ
Assistant Professor, Department of
Physical Medicine and
Rehabilitation
UMDNJ–New Jersey Medical School
Newark, NJ

Nathan Notter, P.T.
Fort Wayne, IN

Jerard H. Pietan, M.D.
Consultant, Department of
Diagnostic Radiology
Mayo Clinic Jacksonville
Jacksonville, FL
Assistant Professor of Radiology
Mayo Medical School
Rochester, MN

Prathima Reddy, M.D.
Resident Physiatrist
Physical Medicine and
 Rehabilitation
William Beaumont Hospital
Royal Oak, MI

Mark V. Reecer, M.D.
Orthopaedics Northeast, P.C.
Fort Wayne, IN

Thomas D. Rizzo, Jr., M.D.
Consultant, Department of Physical
 Medicine and Rehabilitation
Mayo Clinic Jacksonville
Jacksonville, FL
Assistant Professor of Physical
 Medicine and Rehabilitation
Mayo Medical School
Rochester, MN

Boris M. Terebuh, M.D.
Orthopaedics Northeast, P.C.
Fort Wayne, IN

Agnes Soriano Wallbom, M.D.
Assistant Professor
Department of Physical Medicine
 and Rehabilitation
University of Michigan
Ann Arbor, MI

Frank Y. Wei, M.D.
Physical Medicine and
 Rehabilitation
Edina, MN

Jacqueline J. Wertsch, M.D.
Professor of Physical Medicine
 and Rehabilitation
Medical College of Wisconsin
Staff Physician
Zablocki Veterans Affairs
Medical Center
Milwaukee, WI

Thomas S. Whitecloud III, M.D.
Professor and Chairman
Department of Orthopedic Sugery
Chief, Division of Spinal Surgery
Tulane University Medical Center
New Orleans, LA

John I. Williams, M.D.
Orthopaedics Northeast, P.C.
Fort Wayne, IN

Robert E. Windsor, M.D.
Assistant Clinical Professor,
 Emory University
President, Georgia Pain
 Physicians, P.C.
Marietta, Norcross, Forest Park,
 and Calhoun, GA

Jeffrey L. Woodward, M.D., M.S.
MMSc, FACP, LMT, PC
Springfield Physical Medicine
 and Rehabilitation
Springfield, MO

Acknowledgments

The authors would like to express their gratitude to those individuals who have made this textbook possible. I would also like to thank my dedicated nurse, Sue Schilb, R.N., for her tireless support of my work. A sincere thank you is also in order for our excellent staff of medical transcriptionists at Orthopaedics Northeast who worked on this program, including Dawn Wiegmann, Pat Weicker, Joan Burton, Jackie Hickman, Shari Bailey, Mona Andrachik, Debora Buerke, and Cheryl Layton-Riley. The Information Systems Department at Orthopaedics Northeast provided much-needed support as well; and thanks also go to Kate Barton, Kathy Crum, and Laurie Riegel. Most importantly, I would like to thank all of the contributing authors who took the time to write excellent chapters despite their many other obligations.

Bryan D. Kaplansky, M.D

Dedication

To my wife Lynn, and children
Benjamin and Kevin,
with love.

ERRATA

Cat # L1244

Occupational Low Back Pain: Aggressive Nonsurgical Care

Bryan Kaplansky, M.D.

Figure 4.7a page 80. The caption should read:

Lumbar paravertebral sympathetic chain block, from *Management of Peripheral Nerve Problems*, Omer, George Jr. and Spencer, M., Eds., W.B. Saunders Co., Philadelphia, 1980, 44–66. With permission.

Figure 6.12 page 124. The caption should read:

Isolated strengthening to hip extensor muscles.

Figure 6.13 page 125. The caption should read:

Hip abductor strengthening. Note that the abdominal muscles are pretightened to prevent movement through the lumbar spine and isolate strengthening to the hip abductors.

Figures 6.5 through 6.10 are out of order. The order should be:

Figure 6.5 should be Figure 6.10
Figure 6.6 should be Figure 6.9
Figure 6.7 should be Figure 6.5
Figure 6.8 should be Figure 6.6
Figure 6.9 should be Figure 6.7
Figure 6.10 should be Figure 6.8

Contents

part one

Diagnostic

chapter one

Low Back Pain: History and Physical Examination

Howard I. Levy, M.D.

1.1 Overview

This chapter will serve to provide clinicians who treat patients with low back pain a method of performing a thorough history and physical examination to elucidate most of the common and some of the uncommon sources of musculoskeletal low back pain. Medical conditions that can be the source for referred pain, such as an abdominal aortic aneurysm, pelvic disorders, urinary tract abnormalities, gastrointestinal disorders as well as rheumatologic conditions will not be addressed in this chapter. The clinician should be cognizant of these conditions that can lead to referred pain and should incorporate physical examination techniques and laboratory and imaging tests to rule out these conditions.

Although Frymoyer found that up to 85% of low back conditions cannot be diagnosed from the history and physical exam or with diagnostic testing,[12] other studies have sought to determine sources for low back pain by using more specific diagnostic techniques.[1, 27, 33, 34, 36] The history and physical examination must be conducted with the knowledge of the various sources of pain mediators involving the lumbar spine.[40, 43] Although the etiology of the pain may never be discovered due to the rapid spontaneous resolution of most low back pain disorders, a clinician can narrow down diagnoses to a few categories in about 75% of the cases just from the history. When the diagnosis may not be clear based on the physical examination or diagnostic testing, a clinician may still be able to identify the source of apparent nonspecific low back pain when there is an understanding of the structures that cause pain and how that pain is manifested.[13] Despite the often nonspecific nature of low back pain, a physician's goal is always to try to precisely locate the pain generator so that a specific treatment program can be outlined for a specific diagnosis.

1.2 History

The history is the cornerstone for the diagnostic evaluation in a patient with complaints of low back pain or sciatica. The key is to narrow down the diagnosis by carefully structuring the questions and listening intently to the answers. The worst case scenarios or "red flag" diagnoses such as cauda equina syndrome, tumors, fractures, and infection can all be ruled out through the history as will be discussed later. Medical conditions that cause referred pain may be diagnosed and a complete workup should always be pursued vigorously when indicated.

1.2.1 Chief Complaint

The first step of the history and in locating pain generators occurs before talking to the patient. A pain drawing assists in identification of the chief complaint by providing a picture of the pain pattern and location.[22] It can map out symptoms, give the clinician an idea of the character and location of the pain and whether it is physiologic[22] (Figures 1.1 to 1.3). Ransford, Cairns, and Mooney first demonstrated the value of pain drawings in distinguishing true back pain complaints from hysterical symptoms in 1976.[30] Those patients who use more than three modalities on the pain drawing had a high incidence of hypochondriasis or hysteria on the Minnesota Multiphasic Personality Inventory.

The next step in identifying the pain generators is to identify the primary location of the pain. It is generally helpful to ask the patient to place a finger on the single most painful spot.

1.2.2 Inciting Event

The character of symptoms at the onset of complaints is important in the identification of pain generators. Acute pain following high energy trauma such as from a fall from a great height or a motor vehicle accident may herald the possibility of a spinal fracture. A lifting injury causing acute pain may result in a herniated disc or a lumbar strain. Repetitive bending or twisting or prolonged truck driving may cause a gradual onset of pain with crescendoing pain syndromes that may be initiated by degenerative changes in the spine. Patients with spinal arthropathies may present with pain of insidious onset over many years. Spontaneous pain in the elderly may indicate the

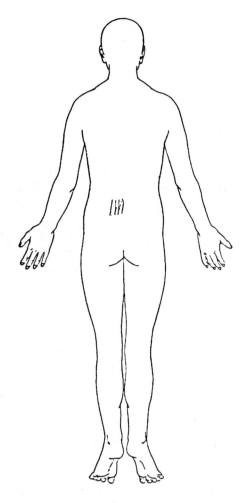

Figure 1.1   Patient drawing of nonradiating low back pain.

presence of spinal metastases. High energy trauma and spontaneous pain in the elderly are red flag indications for performing diagnostic tests sooner than other presentations.

1.2.3   Character and Location of Pain

The next step in locating pain generators once onset has been determined is the current location of the pain and how it has changed since its onset. Additionally it is helpful to determine whether this is an initial or recurrent episode of pain. Disc herniations causing sciatica may begin with intermittent low back pain followed by the onset of predominant leg pain

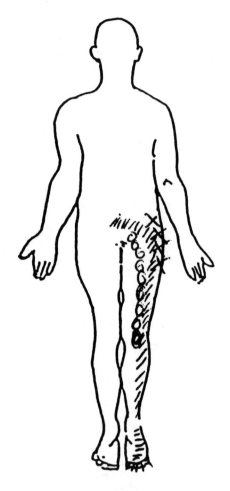

Figure 1.2   Pain drawing by a patient with S1 radiculopathy. O's represent pins and needles, X's represent burning, and /'s represent stabbing.

with little back pain. Whether the pain radiates in a true radicular fashion or the pain is referred in a nondermatomal pattern can be determined by whether there are any associated symptoms aside from pain, such as numbness, weakness, or paresthesias, which may indicate true nerve root compression. In a recurrent episode, clarification of how the pain has changed may signify a different or additional diagnosis.

Positions of relief and aggravation are important clues to diagnosis. Patients with disc herniations have difficulty sitting and are better standing or lying down. Patients with arthritis, sprains, and strains get relief from pain while seated and lying down. Lumbar stenotic patients, on the other hand, get relief when sitting and have a consistent pattern of neurogenic claudication that develops after walking a known distance. Use of a shopping cart may enhance the patient's ability to ambulate.

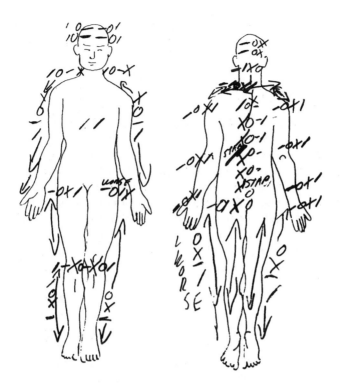

Figure 1.3 Pain drawing by a patient with nonorganic pain syndrome. O's represent pins and needles, X's represent burning, /'s represent stabbing pain, ='s represent numbness, +'s represent throbbing, and → represent aching

1.2.4 Past Spinal Surgical History

A history of prior surgical intervention for a lumbar pain syndrome may provide vital clues to the origin of the current complaints. The relevant history of prior spinal surgery answers the following questions: Did the patient have relief from the surgery? Did the symptoms change after surgery? If the presurgical pain returned, how soon after surgery did it recur? And, how long did it take the patient to recover from the surgery? In addition, it is important to understand what type of prior surgery has been performed. A patient with a simple discectomy presents different problems from one with a prior lumbar fusion.

Patients with no relief from surgery may have had inappropriate surgery. Those with immediate relief after discectomy but recurrent pain shortly thereafter may have had a complication such as a recurrent disc herniation or an infection. Those with relief for approximately six months followed by recurrent symptoms may have epidural scarring. Furthermore, patients with instrumented fusions and chronic or recurrent pain may have symptoms secondary to pseudoarthrosis. It may take time for the instrumentation to become loose following an instrumented fusion as opposed to uninstrumented fusions which may lead to symptoms heralding a pseudoarthrosis sooner. Smoking inhibits fusion from solidifying and thus patients who smoke are at a higher risk for pseudoarthrosis.[39]

1.2.5 Occupational History Issues

Occupational risk factors must be explored during the history. Patients with heavy, demanding work may have an increased risk for back pain. Consequently, questions regarding risk factors associated with work should be taken into consideration. Bending, twisting, or lifting heavy objects repetitively with a bending motion can increase the risk for back pain.[6, 25] Truck drivers and bus drivers are subjected to vibratory stresses to the spine.[19] Vibration has been shown to increase the risk for lumbar disc herniations.[19] Truck drivers also may do heavy lifting, thus having increased risk factors for injury to the lumbar spine.[19] Prolonged sitting, obesity, and smoking may also be associated with increased incidence of low back pain and HNP.[6, 14, 15]

Psychosocial issues also must be considered when examining occupational risk factors.[9, 13, 23, 26] People who are unhappy or dissatisfied with their jobs, supervisors, or compensation may be at increased risk for low back pain.[2, 4, 14, 21, 27, 29] Additionally, any connection with the Workers' Compensation system or lawsuits is associated with disability secondary to back pain. Studies have shown that patients involved with lawsuits related to back pain causation have a poorer prognosis for recovery.[23, 37]

1.2.6 Tumors, Infections, Fractures, and Cauda Equina Syndrome

The next phase of the history is to rule out several of the worst-case scenario diagnoses which are tumor, infection, fracture, and cauda equina syndrome.

The diagnosis of *cauda equina syndrome,* a progressive neurologic deficit in a patient with low back pain and sciatica, must be ruled out first. This diagnosis, although rare, is a surgical emergency. Patient complaints include urinary retention with overflow incontinence, bilateral sciatica, "saddle anesthesia," difficulty with walking and a loss of control of the lower extremities. Magnetic resonance imaging confirms or eliminates this diagnosis. Immediate referral to a spine surgeon is of paramount importance.

The possibility that a patient has a tumor should also always be addressed. Deyo et al.[5] has shown that a tumor should be considered in a patient over the age of 50 with a history of unremitting symptoms despite conservative care, and a disturbance of sleep due to pain. The patient's pain is not relieved by rest or change in position. A history of unexplained weight loss and a previous history of cancer are also important indicators. Patients with a history of breast cancer, lung cancer, or prostate cancer are at risk for spinal metastases. Extra spinal causes for low back pain and leg pain may be due to tumors (Figure 1.4).

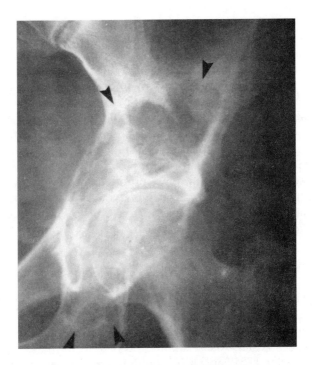

Figure 1.4   Pelvic tumor in patient with low back and lower limb pain.

Symptoms of fever, chills, or night sweats may indicate a spinal infection in patients with back pain.[31] A previous history of an infection such as a urinary tract infection, a skin infection, or i.v. drug abuse are risk factors.[7] The patient must be asked if he or she has an illness that predisposes him or her to infection. Is he or she immunocompromised? The patient may also complain of sleep disturbance similar to those patients with tumors. Percussion tenderness over the spinous process in these patients may help direct the physician to the diagnosis of osteomyelitis or discitis.

Spinal fractures in younger patients are rare. Fractures may occur after high-energy trauma. Most of these patients are seen in an emergency room initially. However some fractures are missed and careful evaluation is always indicated. The historical details and pain complaints may not provide sufficient information for the practitioner to differentiate benign sprains from neurologically threatening fractures; thus examination and appropriate diagnostic testing for persistent pain complaints after high energy trauma may be indicated. Compression fractures may occur spontaneously in elderly patients or in those patients on chronic steroid medication, without significant trauma.

1.3   Physical Exam

The physical exam expands the understanding of the source of the patient's pain. It is an extension of the history.

1.3.1   Observation

Examination of the patient with low back pain starts with the entry of the patient. The clinician should document antalgic gait patterns and if the patient is exhibiting any signs of pain.[18] Any unusual methods of transfer should be documented along with any signs of discomfort while the patient is sitting. Unusual pain behavior that would not be consistent with a diagnosis found through the history or physical exam should be documented.

After the initial observation of the patient, the physical examination is divided into three phases characterized by the position of the patient: 1) standing; 2) seated; and 3) lying down on the exam table sequentially in prone, supine, and lateral decubitus positions. In this way the patient's pain complaint can be observed, and reactions to physical testing can be observed in both loaded and unloaded positions.

1.3.2   Standing Phase

The patient should stand with his back to the clinician while being examined initially. Document any superficial skin lesions that may indicate underlying spine pathology. There should be an examination for rashes, such as that seen with herpes zoster. Also examine the patient for abnormalities in posture such as a lateral shift and pelvic obliquity. Symmetry of the arm positions at rest should be noted. Asymmetry may indicate scoliosis. Skin-fold asymmetry may also be indicative of a scoliotic curve. Check for shoulder girdle asymmetry and scapular winging. Observe from a lateral view the lumbar lordosis and its relationship to thoracic kyphosis and cervical lordosis. The level of the anterior superior iliac spine can be assessed. The level of the shoulders and hips can be assessed and a plumb-bob can be dropped from C-7 to ensure that there is proper balance in the sagittal plane (Figure 1.5).

Palpation over the lumbar spine to identify tender points is the next step. Tenderness over the PSIS may indicate SI joint symptoms or cluneal nerve irritation. Fatty nodules that may become painful can be palpated. Bony prominences that are painful to palpation or percussion can help identify fractures, tumors or infections.

A *Schober's test* can be performed to measure the degree of restriction of spine/forward flexion by placing the thumb at the lumbosacral junction with the fingers approximately 10 cm above (Figure 1.6). The patient then flexes the lumbar spine. The examiner looks for the excursion distance between the thumb and the finger that is placed above (Figure 1.7). Distances of less than an additional 5 cm would be considered abnormal. Any rib humps indicative of scoliosis can be observed when the patient is fully flexed. A rib hump on the right is consistent with idiopathic scoliosis. A rib hump on the left is possibly an indicator for other disorders and requires an in-depth work up.

The patient's reaction to directional range of motion should be recorded. The rhythm of forward and lateral flexion, rotation, and extension is ob-

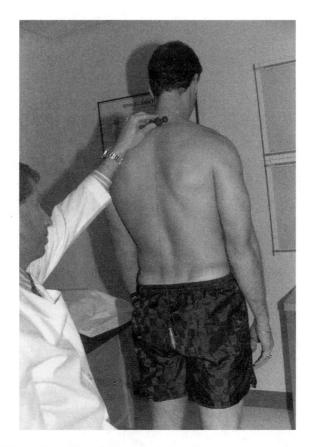

Figure 1.5   Plumb-bob utilized to assess alignment.

served. Patients with low back and lower limb pain with forward flexion may have a discogenic and radicular source for their symptoms. Those individuals with low back and lower limb pain with lumbar extension and extension rotation may have a component of lumbar spinal stenosis with radiculopathy. However, patients with mechanical low back pain can have similar symptoms for the low back and lower limb with range of motion due to referred pain from structures such as the sacroiliac and facet joints.

1.3.3   Seated Phase

Strength, reflexes and sensation can be tested while the patient is seated. Motor, sensory, or reflex changes should be examined to identify nerve root abnormalities. The most common roots involved are L5, S1, and L4. The L5 root sensory distribution is over the lateral aspect of the calf, the dorsum of the foot, and the first web space. Reflex changes are not commonly found but can be seen with the hamstrings. Muscle weakness of the extensor hallucis

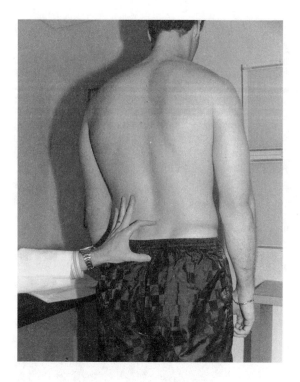

Figure 1.6 Schober's test.

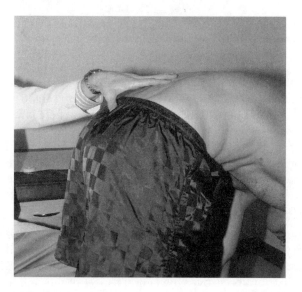

Figures 1.7   Schober's test.

longus which is predominantly L5 can be identified. The S1 root has sensation along the posterior calf to the lateral aspect of the foot and heel. Motor power can be assessed by asking the patient to fatigue the gastroc soleus muscle group by standing on the toes. The L4 root sensation is anteromedial on the leg down to the instep of the foot. The quadriceps reflex is L4 and motor function can be assessed by the tibialis anterior and quadriceps.

A *seated straight leg flip test* allows the clinician to check the reliability of the supine straight leg raise test when done surreptitiously (Figure 1.8). The patient can be led to believe that the physician is checking for peripheral pulses or sensations or some other test while the leg is extended. Discrepancy between the seated test and the supine test may indicate a patient is malingering. This is also a good time to perform the *slump test* by having the patient flex his neck and torso (Figure 1.9). This accentuates any neural impingement such as secondary to a herniated disc, by further stretching the nerve root.

Cervical spine range of motion should be addressed in patients with lower limb pain. A cervical myelopathy can lead to lower limb symptoms, although this is uncommon without other associated myelopathic complaints.

1.3.4 Supine Phase

In the supine position a positive *straight leg raise test* leads to pain radiating from the lower back, through the buttocks and down past the knee. In reporting a straight leg test, the degree at which the patient feels pain and the

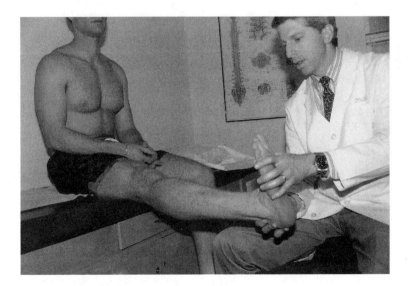

Figure 1.8   Seated straight leg flip test.

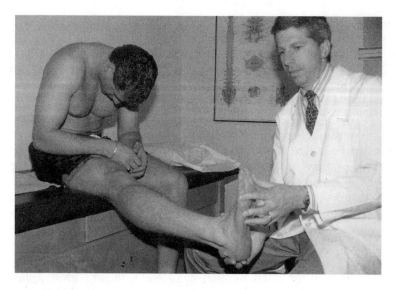

Figure 1.9 Slump test.

distribution of the symptoms should be indicated. Pain at less than 30 degrees (Figure 1.10) or greater than 70 degrees may indicate an unreliable
test.[10, 38] Figure 1.11 demonstrates a straight leg raise of approximately 45 degrees; this coupled with consistent leg pain below the knee is a positive test.
A supine straight leg raise with pain at less than 30 degrees and a seated
straight leg test that is negative may indicate secondary gain or nonorganic

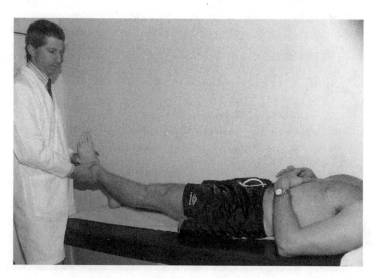

Figure 1.10 Supine straight leg raise test with symptoms elicited at less than
30 degrees.

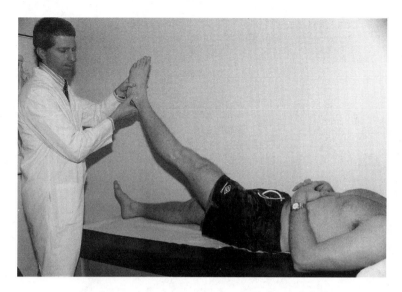

Figure 1.11 Supine straight leg raise test with symptoms elicited at 45 degrees.

issues. The *contralateral* or *cross straight leg raising test* involves elevating the uninvolved limb. A positive test causes pain into the opposite side which is the patient's symptomatic limb.

Patrick's maneuver (Figure 1.12) and Gaenslen's test (Figure 1.13) are commonly utilized to test for sacroiliac joint dysfunction. *Patrick's maneuver* is done with the hip flexed, abducted, and externally rotated in a figure of four. Pressure may be placed on the contralateral side of the pelvis. Groin pain may indicate hip pathology; back pain in the sacroiliac joint region may be consistent with sacroiliac pain. The *Gaenslen's test* is performed by having the patient slide to the edge of the table until the buttock is partially hanging off the table. The lower limb is allowed to drop off the table into extension and a small amount of stress is placed over the anterior thigh while holding the opposite limb in flexion to stress the sacroiliac joint. Pain in a familiar pattern over the sacroiliac joint is a positive test.

Hip, knee, and ankle range of motion is checked to eliminate any joint sources that may mimic sciatica. Palpation over the greater trochanteric bursa and the iliotibial band may provide clues to extraspinal sources for limb pain. Tinel's sign can be elicited by tapping the peroneal nerve as it crosses the fibular head. The lateral femoral cutaneous nerve can be palpated at the inguinal ligament to elicit thigh paresthesias and pain consistent with meralgia paresthetica. The tarsal tunnel and plantar nerves can be evaluated as a possible source for foot symptoms. Limb atrophy and limb length discrepancies should be noted. Limb pulses, swelling, discoloration, temperature asymmetry, and skin appearance should be recorded.

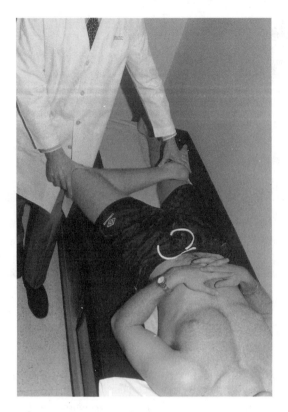

Figure 1.12 Patrick's maneuver.

An examination of the chest wall and abdomen should be undertaken to rule out nonspinal sources for back pain such as rib fractures or an abdominal aortic aneurysm.

1.3.5 Prone Phase

The spinous processes and the soft tissues can be palpated in the prone position. The *sacroiliac shear test* may be performed by placing the hand over a patient's coccygeal region and another hand over the iliac wing with the stress being straight across that plane (Figure 1.14). The test may also be performed by placing one hand underneath the ischium and another hand on top of the sacrum. By compressing the joint in that manner, the patient may feel familiar pain. Tenderness can be elicited in the sciatic notch.

Patients can be tested for piriformis syndrome by placing them in a side-lying position, flexing the hip and knee, and then allowing the hip to be abducted and internally rotated. By palpating in the buttock and along the edge of the posterior inferior aspect of the greater trochanter, piriformis tenderness may be elicited by palpation of the end of the piriformis muscle. Some

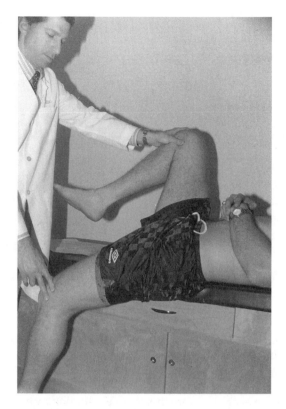

Figure 1.13   Gaenslen's test.

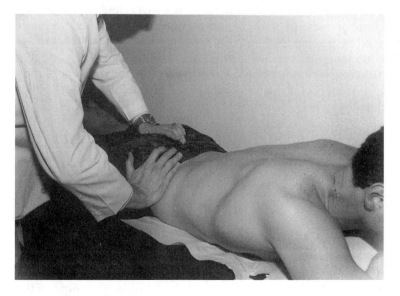

Figure 1.14   Sacroiliac shear test.

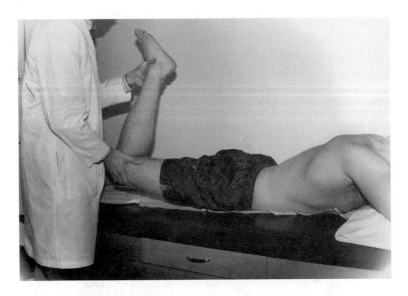

Figure 1.15   Femoral stretch sign.

physicians have recommended a vaginal or rectal exam to palpate the piriformis muscle inside the sacrum. The genitourinary and rectal exams may also be necessary to rule out pathologic intrapelvic sources of pain in certain individuals. If such a condition is suspected or if other nonmusculoskeletal abnormalities are possible, a more thorough evaluation by a family physician or internist is recommended.

In the prone position, the *femoral stretch sign* (Figure 1.15) may indicate upper lumbar radiculopathy or more peripheral neural compromise. It is performed by placing the hand under the patient's distal femur and extending the hip joint. Patients will complain of pain in the anterior thigh region. When the patient sits with one knee up to the chest to take some of the stretch off of the nerve root, it may indicate an upper lumbar disc herniation with radiculopathy.

1.4   Specific Syndromes with Findings on History and Physical Exam

Following a thorough history and physical exam, a diagnosis of most of the syndromes associated with low back pain can be made without using any expensive or invasive diagnostic workups. A few patients will require specific diagnostic tests which will be discussed at greater length in future chapters.

1.4.1   Discogenic Low Back Pain

Discogenic low back pain is defined as back pain due to lesions of the disc.[8] The lesions include internal disc disruption, annular tears, and contained and uncontained disc herniations that result in low back pain without sciatica.[8] Historically patients with discogenic low back pain complain of difficulty in sitting, particularly sitting at a desk or driving a car. Symptoms may have been intermittent for years with occasional exacerbations. Standing and stretching into lumbar extension may relieve the pain. Valsalva maneuvers such as bowel movements, coughing, or sneezing may exacerbate the pain. The *bilateral active straight leg raise*[42] may produce excruciating low back pain. During palpation, the clinician may be able to identify the level that is painful with compression over the spinous processes.

1.4.2 Herniated Nucleus Pulposus with Sciatica

Lumbar disc herniations that cause sciatica can be distinguished from discogenic low back pain. Patients with sciatica complain about pain radiating down the leg to the foot. The patient with sciatica will often have pain radiating to the foot during supine and seated straight leg raise testing.[24] This can be confirmed with the *Lasegue* maneuver where the limb is dropped several degrees from the point of pain radiating down the leg which will then relieve the pain; when the ankle is dorsiflexed it may re-exacerbate the leg pain. Palpation of the posterior popliteal space may exacerbate leg pain which with the associated neurologic findings of numbness, weakness and pain, is called a *bowstring sign*. Patients with a radiculopathy will also present with specific neurological deficits based on the nerve root level involved (Table 1.1).

1.4.3 Sacroiliac Joint Dysfunction

The sacroiliac joint has been implicated in nonspecific low back pain.[1, 32] The standard teaching in most orthopaedic texts has been that this joint could not be a source for any significant amount of pain, but recently studies have shown that the sacroiliac joint can be a mediator for significant pain and indeed can mimic sciatica.[1, 11, 32] Through diagnosis with intraarticular injections using fluoroscopic guidance as the "gold standard," approximately 30% of those patients with previously diagnosed nonspecific chronic back pain were found to have sacroiliac joint dysfunction as the pain mediator.[32]

Table 1. Neurological deficits for common lumbosacral radiculopathies

Nerve root	Strength	Sensation	Reflexes
L4	Ankle dorsiflexion	Anteromedial leg and medial foot	Patellar reflex
L5	Great toe extension	Lateral leg and dorsal foot	Hamstrings
S1	Ankle plantarflexion	Posterior leg and heel/lateral foot	Achilles reflex

Although some studies have reported that sacroiliac joint abnormalities can be identified and diagnosed through a series of simple provocative maneuvers,[20] others have shown that no physical examination technique or provocative maneuver can reliably diagnose patients as having sacroiliac joint pain.[18, 19]

1.4.4   Facet Joint Dysfunction

Facet joint dysfunction is a potential source for low back pain. Studies utilizing fluoroscopically guided diagnostic facet joint injections have reported that some patients with a previous diagnosis of nonspecific low back pain have pain generated from the facet joints.[34, 36] This source of pain though may not be clearly elucidated by simple history and physical exam techniques.[34–36]

1.4.5   Soft Tissue and Ligamentous Low Back Pain

Soft tissue and ligamentous sources for pain are more difficult to diagnose but fortunately most of these patients with this diagnosis will result in relatively benign conditions that will resolve spontaneously. Once other types of diagnoses are ruled out, musculoligamentous or musculotendinous disorders can be considered a diagnosis of exclusion.

1.4.6   Lumbar Spinal Stenosis

In lumbar spinal stenosis, another source for leg pain, the history may provide more clues than the physical exam.[17] Neurogenic claudication is the hallmark for lumbar spinal stenosis.[17] It is leg pain from what may be a local vascular phenomenon causing ischemia to the nerves resulting in leg pain. A history of leaning over a shopping cart for relief while walking may suggest the diagnosis of lumbar spinal stenosis, since flexion tends to relieve the radicular symptoms from stenosis.

1.4.7   Spondylolysis, Spondylolisthesis, and Instability

Spondylolysis and spondylolisthesis cannot be clearly diagnosed from the findings of the history and physical examination. To diagnose these entities, imaging studies are necessary although the history and physical exam provide clues as to whether the imaging study findings are clinically relevant. A patient with spondylolisthesis may have had an insidious pattern of pain that has persisted for many years prior to a work injury. This insidious pattern may be indicative of intermittent irritation in the area of the spondylolisthesis. The issue of physical findings is a bit more complex. One study examining the clinical findings in patients with spondylolysis and spondylolisthesis demonstrated that the physical examination may be normal in a mild spondylolysis or a mild spondylolisthesis.[31] Patients may have tightness of the hamstrings or a peculiar gait pattern. A "step-off" may be palpated for the spinous processes; however this is not clearly found except in high-grade spondylolisthesis. Symptoms may begin in younger patients with back and buttock pain being the most frequent findings with occasional radicular pain.[3, 16] Neurological deficits such as reflex abnormalities, atrophy and weakness may be noted in only approximately 35% of patients.

1.4.8 Nonorganic Back Pain

Psychosocial issues may complicate occupational low back pain disorders. A patient's occupational injury report may have historical details that can assist the physician in assessing if there are concurrent psychological or secondary gain issues. These patients may have a pain level out of character to their observed behavior. Waddell and colleagues have developed a simple set of specific tests to help determine the presence of nonorganicity associated with occupational back pain (Table 1.2).[41] Examples of tests that may elicit pain complaints include superficial tenderness with light touch over the skin that involves a wide area of the lumbar spine, low back pain with axial loading on the top of the head, and simulated rotation of the spine by holding the patient's hips and rotating the pelvis instead of the spine. The discrepancy between seated and supine straight leg raising, sensory disturbances that are not characteristic of a specific dermatomal or root pattern, and "giving way" type weakness, as well as overreaction during the physical examination are other examples of Waddell signs. Three or more of these signs may indicate that the patient has nonorganic pain behavior. The presence of nonorganicity should be clearly elucidated prior to embarking on any

Table 1.2 Waddell Signs

*Tenderness
Superficial
Nonanatomic

*Simulation Tests
Axial loading
Rotation

*Regional Disturbances
Weakness
Sensory

*Overreaction

*Distraction Tests
Straight leg raising

expensive testing and treatment and certainly in those patients who are considered candidates for surgery.

1.5 Summary

The evaluation of occupational low back pain poses a challenge to physicians. Although most cases of low back pain may be nonspecific and it may be difficult to precisely diagnose a specific source for the pain, a careful history, and a physical examination should allow the clinician to rule out the more serious causes of back pain and broadly categorize the potential pain generator in the majority of individuals. The history and physical exam is the first and most important step in the evaluation process. It allows the clinician to determine the necessity for proceeding with imaging, electrodiagnostic, and laboratory tests. The findings on the history and physical provide the framework for treatment. The more specific the diagnosis, the more specific and appropriate the treatment program becomes which should pave the way for cost-effective treatment with better outcomes.

1.6 References

1. Bernard, T. N., Kirkaldy-Willis, W. H. Recognizing specific characteristics of nonspecific low back pain. *Clin. Orthop.* 217:266–280, 1987.
2. Bigos, S. J., Battie, M. C., Spengler, D. M. A prospective study of work perceptions and psychosocial factors affecting the report of back injury. *Spine* 16:1–6, 1991.
3. Boxall, D., Bradford, D. S., Winter, R. B. et al. Management of severe spondylolisthesis in children and adolescents. *J. Bone Joint Surg.* 61-A:479–495, 1979.
4. Deyo, R. A. Occupational back pain. State of the Art Review. *Spine* 2:7–30, 1987.
5. Deyo, R. A., Diehi, A. K. Cancer as a cause of back pain: Frequency, clinical presentation and diagnostic strategies. *J. Intern. Med.* 3:230–238, 1988.
6. Deyo, R. A., Loeser, J. D., Bigos, S. J. Herniated lumbar intervertebral disk. *Ann. Intern. Med.* 112:598–603, 1997.
7. Deyo, R. A., Rainville, J., Kent, D. L. What can the history and physical examination tell us about low back pain? *JAMA* 268:760–765, 1997.
8. Dvorak, J., Dvorak, V. *Manual Medicine Diagnostics.* New York: Thieme-Stratton, 1984.
9. Eastrarid, N. Medical, psychological, and social factors associated with back abnormalities, and self reported back pain: A cross sectional study of male employees in a Swedish pulp and paper industry. *Br. J. Ind. Med.* 44:327–336, 1987.
10. Fahmi, W. H. Observations on straight leg raising with special reference to nerve root adhesions. *Can. J. Surg.* 9:44–48, 1970.
11. Fortin, J. D., Dwyer, A. P., West, S. et al. Sacroiliac joint: Pain referral maps upon applying a new injection arthrography technique. Part I: Asymptomatic volunteers. *Spine* 19:1475–1482, 1994.
12. Frymoyer, J. W. Back pain and sciatica. *N. Engl. J. Med.* 318:291–300, 1988.

13. Frymoyer, J. W., Rosen, J. C., Clements, J. H. et al. Psychologic factors in low-back pain disability. *Clin. Orthop.* 195:178–184, 1985.
14. Hanley, E. N., Shapiro, D. E. The development of low-back pain after excision of a lumbar disc. *J. Bone Joint Surg.* 71-A:719–721, 1989.
15. Heliovarra, M. Body height, obesity, and risk of herniated lumbar interverte-bral disc. *Spine* 12:469–472, 1987.
16. Hensinger, R. N. Spondylolysis and spondylolisthesis in children and adoles-cents. *J. Bone Joint Surg.* 71-A:1098–1107, 1989.
17. Katz, J. N., Dalgas, M., Stack, G. et al. Degenerative lumbar spinal stenosis: Diagnostic value of the history and physical examination. *Arthritis Rheum.* 38:1236–1241, 1995.
18. Keek, F. J., Wilkins, R. H., Cook, W. A. Direct observation of pain behavior in low back pain patients during physical examination. *Pain* 20:59–68, 1984.
19. Kelsey, J. L., Githens, P. B., O'Connor, T. et al. Acute prolapsed lumbar interver-tebral disc. An epidemiologic study with special reference to driving automo-biles and cigarette smoking. *Spine* 9:608–613, 1984.
20. Laslett, M.,Williams, M. The reliability of selected pain provocation tests for sacroiliac joint pathology. *Spine* 19:1243–1249, 1994.
21. Linton, S. J., Wang, L. E. Attributions (beliefs) and job satisfaction associated with back pain in an industrial setting. *Percept. Mot. Skills* 76:51–62, 1993.
22. Mann, N. H., Brown, M. D., Hertz, D. B. et al. Initial impression diagnosis using low-back pain patient pain drawings. *Spine* 18:41–53, 1993.
23. Milhous, R. L., Haugh, L. D., Frymoyer, J. W. et al. Determinants of vocational disability in patients with low back pain. *Pain Arch. P. M. & R.* 70:589–593, 1989.
24. Morris, E. W., Di Paola, M., Vallance, R. et al. G. Diagnosis and decision making in lumbar disc prolapse and nerve entrapment. *Spine* 11:436–439, 1986.
25. Mundt, D. J., Kelsey, J. L., Golden, A. L. et al. An Epidemiologic study of nonoccupational lifting as a risk factor for herniated lumbar intervertebral disc. *Spine* 18:595–602, 1993.
26. Nachemson, A. L. Newest knowledge of low back pain: A critical look. *Clin. Orthop.* 279:8–20, 1992.
27. Nehemkis, A., Carver, O. W., Evanski, P. M. The predictive utility of the ortho-pedic examination in identifying the low back pain patient with hysterical per-sonality features. *Clin. Orthop.* 145:158–162, 1979.
28. Nice, D. A., Riddle, D. L., Lamb, R. L. et al. Intertester reliability of judgments of the presence of trigger points in patients with low back pain. *Arch. Phys. Med. Rehabil.* 73:893–898, 1992.
29. Pope, M. H., Rosen, J. C., Wilder, D. G. et al. The relation between biomechanical and psychological factors in patients with low back pain. *Spine* 5:173, 1980.
30. Ransford, A. O., Cairns, D., Mooney, V. The pain drawing as an aid to the psy-chological evaluation of patients with low back pain. *Spine* 1:127–134, 1976.
31. Sapico, F. L., Montgomerie, J. Z. Vertebral osteomyelitis. (Review). *Infect. Dis. Clin. North Am.* 4:539–550, 1990.
32. Schwarzer, A. C., Aprill, C. N., Bogduk, N. The sacroiliac joint in chronic low back pain. *Spine* 20:31–37, 1995.
33. Schwarzer, A. C., Aprill, C. N., Derby, R. et al. The prevalence and clinical fea-tures of internal disc disruption in patients with chronic low back pain. *Spine* 20:1878–1883, 1995.

34. Schwarzer, A. C., Derby, R., Aprill, C. et al. Pain from the lumbar zygapophysial joints: A test of two models. *J. Spinal Disorders* 7:331–336, 1994.
35. Schwarzer, A. C., Derby, R., Aprill, C. N. et al. The value of the provocation response in lumbar zygapophysial joint injections. *Clin. J. Pain* 10:309–313, 1994.
36. Schwarzer, A. C., Wang, S. C., O'Driscoll, D. et al. The ability of computed tomography to identify a painful zygapophysial joint in patients with chronic low back pain. *Spine* 20:907–912, 1995.
37. Seres, J. L., Newman, R. I. Negative influences of the disability compensation system: Perspectives for the clinician. *Semin. Neurol.* 3:360–369, 1983.
38. Shiging, X., Quanzhi, Z., Dehao, F. et al. Significance of the straight-leg-raising test in the diagnosis and clinic evaluation of lower lumbar intervertebral-disc protrusions. *Bone Joint Surg.* 69-A:517–522, 1987.
39. Silcox III, D. H., Daftari, T., Boden, S. D. et al. The effect of nicotine on spinal fusion. *Spine* 20:1549–1553, 1995.
40. Van den Hougan, H. M. M., Koes, B. W., van Eijk, J. T. M. et al. On the accuracy of history, physical examination, and leukocyte sedimentation rate in diagnosing low back pain in general practice: A criteria-based review of the literature. *Spine* 20:318–327, 1995.
41. Waddell, G., Mulloch, J. A., Kunmel, E. et al. Nonorganic physical signs in low back pain. *Spine* 5:117–125, 1980.
42. Waddell, G. W., Somerville, M. B., Huverson, I. et al. Objective clinical evaluation of physical Impairment in chronic low back pain. *Spine* 17:617–628, 1992.
43. White III, M., Gordon, S. L. Synopsis: Workshop on idiopathic low back pain. *Spine* 7:141–149, 1982.

chapter two

The Appropriate Utilization of Imaging Studies for Disorders of the Lumbar Spine

Thomas D. Rizzo, Jr., M.D.
Jerard H. Pietan, M.D.
Mark V. Reecer, M.D.

2.1 Overview

When treating lumbar spine injuries, imaging studies frequently provide valuable information that facilitates patient management and confirms the diagnosis. The use of these studies is often expected by the patient at the time of their initial evaluation. However, the studies that are available do have inherent limitations and are associated with false positive findings. A detailed history and physical examination will provide the information necessary to formulate a detailed plan for treatment and evaluation. The use of imaging studies is based upon this information. The judicious choice of these studies will reduce costs and also reduce the likelihood of making an incorrect diagnosis. Tests are often ordered based upon nonspecific subjective complaints, without substantiating objective findings on physical examinations. This was demonstrated when compensated workers with back pain and leg pain were shown to be twice as likely to have a negative CT or myelogram as noncompensated patients.[1]

2.2   Role of Imaging in Low Back Pain

Studies evaluating the use of imaging modalities look predominantly at their relative cost, and whether they can identity a given abnormality. Attempts are made to compare a given imaging study with the "gold standard" test for back pain. This criteria may be appropriate for most diseases however, low back pain does not fit the traditional pathology model. As physicians, we are often frustrated by this and continue on an often endless search for the "pain generator," despite the fact that treatment is not necessarily affected by these studies. This is particularly true considering that common muscle and ligamentous injuries of the spine do not normally show abnormalities on imaging studies. Therefore, this frequently encountered cause of back pain is diagnosed based upon the clinical presentation and examination, not on imaging studies.

Inherent weaknesses in these studies may lead to an overestimation of the diagnostic accuracy and the value of imaging technology. The technology has to be evaluated in light of its clinical impact.[2] Simply put, an imaging study does not diagnose a condition, the physician does. The imaging study provides a valuable piece of information, but this information does not exist independently of the clinical picture or the physician's judgment. There were no studies between 1985 and 1995 that looked at the therapeutic implications of test results and there were few that correlated imaging study results with patient outcomes.[2]

A variety of studies have determined that the cost for caring for an injured worker is twice as much as for a nonworker.[3-7] It is not clear whether this increase in cost is related to the prices charged[3-4] or because services are overutilized.[3, 5, 7]

In several studies that looked at the patterns of physicians ordering diagnostic studies, accepted guidelines for ordering were not followed, expensive imaging tests were over-ordered, and specialists were over-consulted. In these same studies, indicated testing and consultations were not performed on some patients who met guidelines for such testing or referrals.[8-10] If guidelines had been followed precisely, some areas of evaluation (e.g., plain radiographs) would have increased. Other studies show that guidelines will decrease the overutilization of some tests, but that this will be offset by the standard ordering of other tests. This may lead to a neutral financial impact.[11] If costs are to be cut, changes in the accepted guidelines have to occur.

One service that was looked at specifically was the utilization of magnetic resonance imaging (MRI) by physicians that owned MRI facilities. Their ordering was compared to the utilization of this imaging modality by physicians that did not have a financial interest in the imaging center.[7] This study found that 28% of MRIs ordered by physicians with a financial stake in an MRI facility were deemed inappropriate.

When considering the direct and indirect costs associated with an injured worker, the diagnostic imaging portion of these costs is certainly not prohibitive. A program at Johns Hopkins has shown that overall Workers' Compensation costs can decline even with an increase in the ordering of tests and imaging studies.[12] This was accomplished by being strict about disability determinations and promptly returning employees to work.

Communication with the radiologist is important in helping to establish the diagnosis or in determining the correct test to order.[13] At one time, clinicians took the approach that the radiologist should be able to provide a diagnosis in the absence of any historical background. Today, with cost containment and a rapid diagnosis being the goal, clinicians and radiologists need to work as a team to develop an appropriate diagnostic plan which minimizes redundant and wasteful testing. Furthermore, historical information can assist the radiologist in reaching an accurate diagnosis.

2.3 Roentgenographs

Plain films are typically taken as anterior-posterior (AP), lateral, and spot images (Figures 2.1a-2.1c). These views are taken with the patient lying down, and therefore are unable to provide information on posture, leg

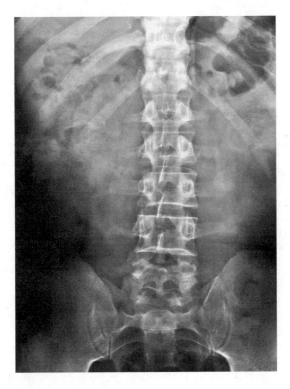

Figure 2.1a AP X-ray of lumbar spine.

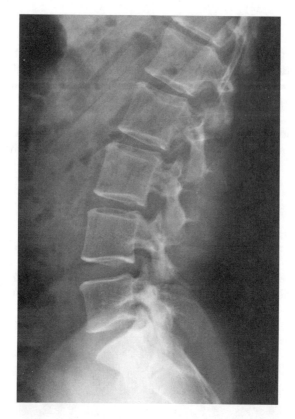

Figure 2.1b   Lateral X-ray of lumbar spine.

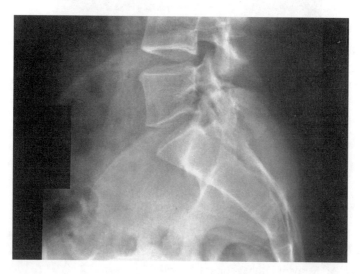

Figure 2.1c   Spot X-ray of lumbar spine.

length, lumbar lordosis, or segmental alignment. Lumbar X-rays are frequently ordered in the setting of low back pain. They are a low cost and noninvasive way of imaging the bony elements of the spine. However, Scavone reported that approximately 75% of lumbar X-rays made no significant impact on treatment decisions.[14] Although limited, these studies also expose the patient to radiation. Considering this, it is important to be judicious when ordering these studies.

Plain films are not typically recommended in the initial 4 weeks following the onset of pain unless specific red flags are identified.[15] Recommended indications or red flags for X-rays in the acute setting include significant trauma, fever, unexplained weight loss, prior cancer, osteoporosis, prolonged steroid use, and IV drug abuse. Traumatic findings may include compression fractures of the vertebral bodies, avulsion fractures, or traumatic fractures to the spinous or transverse processes. (Figure 2.2, and 2.3) Along with the above indications, Deyo suggested X-rays in patients over age 50, with pending litigation or Workers' Compensation proceedings, or neuromuscular deficits.[16]

AP views are taken from the front to the back, and can show angulation secondary to trauma to the lateral aspect of the vertebral bodies (Figure 2.4). This can also provide a look at the pedicles and the facet joints, although the facets are better visualized on oblique views. Abnormalities of the pedicles are more likely due to destructive lesions rather than traumatic injuries.

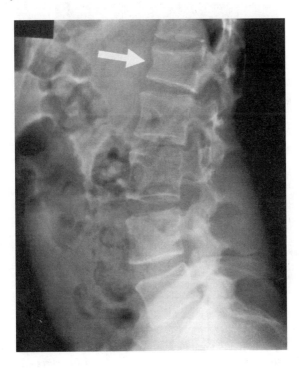

Figure 2.2 L1 vertebral body compression fracture (arrow).

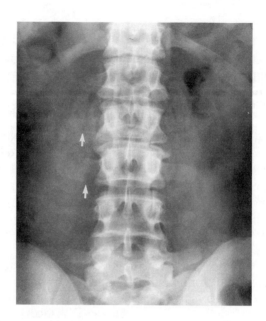

Figure 2.3   Right L2 and L3 transverse process fractures (arrows).

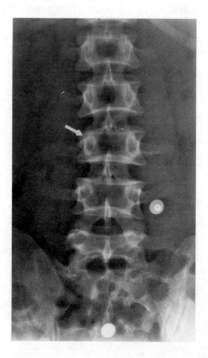

Figure 2.4   AP view of L3 vertebral body compression fracture. From Berquist, Thomas H., *Imaging Atlas of Orthopedic Appliances and Prostheses*, New York: Raven Press, 1995. With permission.

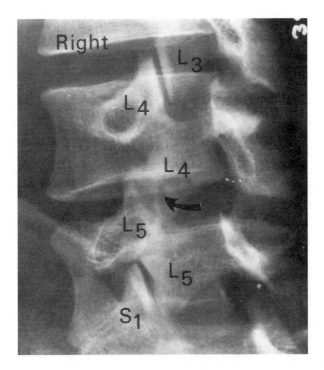

Figure 2.5   Oblique X-rays show L4–5 facet joint arthrosis. From Berquist, Thomas H., *Imaging of Orthopedic Trauma and Surgery*, Philadelphia: W. B. Saunders and Co., 1986. With permission.

Oblique views of the lumbar spine help to visualize the pars inter-articularis — the bony body between the superior and inferior facets of a particular vertebrae. This view also looks down the facet joint and can be an option in documenting arthrosis in this joint. Facet arthrosis (Figure 2.5) can be a source of pain. But it is in assessing the pars interarticularis that this view is most useful. This view has the appearance of the "scottie dog." This is visualized with the pedicle forming the eye of the dog, the inferior articular facet forming the front leg, the superior articular facet is the ear, the transverse process is the nose, and the pars interarticularis is the neck of the dog. A fracture of the pars, or spondylolysis, is seen as a disruption in the "neck of the dog" (Figure 2.6). These views are not obtained routinely, but are very helpful when assessing the posterior elements of the spinal column. However, Rhea reported only 2% of oblique views provided additional information that changed their radiographic interpretation.[17]

With evidence of a pars defect or spondylolisthesis (Figure 2.7) one should consider flexion and extension views. These films help to determine if there is any instability between vertebral segments (Figure 2.8a, b). Motion studies are not necessary unless there is historical data or physical

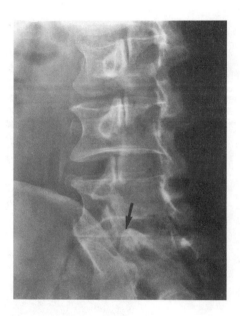

Figure 2.6   Lumbar pars interarticularis fracture (arrow) From Berquist, Thomas H., *Imaging Atlas of Orthopedic Appliances and Prostheses*, New York: Raven Press, 1995. With permission.

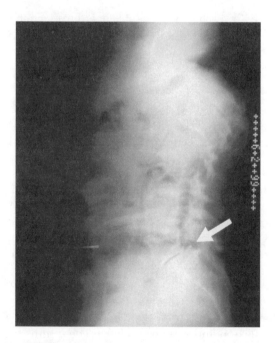

Figure 2.7   Lateral X-rays show L5-S1 spondylolisthesis with marked disc space narrowing (arrow).

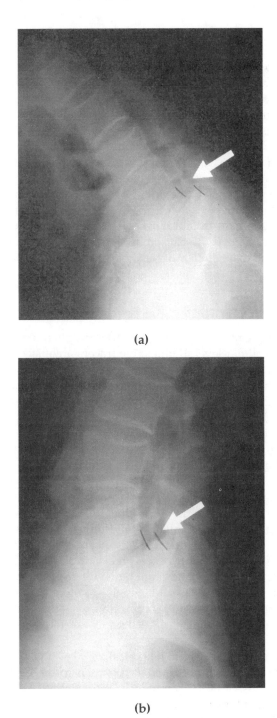

(a)

(b)

Figure 2.8a, b   Instability on lateral flexion (a) and extension (b) X-rays (parallel lines).

findings to suggest instability that can come from instability. There is disagreement as to the radiographic definition of instability, with Boden defining this as >3.5 mm of horizontal translation on a lateral weight-bearing radiograph.[18] This radiographic method though may provide a false negative conclusion.[2] These views may be compromised by significant pain or paraspinal spasms which can limit range of motion, thus reducing the likelihood of demonstrating excessive motion. Other signs or symptoms that would prompt obtaining these views would include an asymmetric appearance to the distance between the spinous processes on the lateral view, along with transient neurologic symptoms on movement.

Side flexion views look at the orientation of the facet joints and how they relate to each other with movement. Spasm and muscle tightness may restrict motion in the absence of structural limitations. Lateral instability is not likely to occur unless the injury was caused by significant trauma. Therefore, these views do not need to be done routinely.

2.4 Bone Scintigraphy

Unlike plain X-rays, nuclear imaging provides insight into the dynamic quality of bone at a cellular level. Radioactive tracers are injected into the blood stream and are taken up by osseous structures that are actively being rebuilt. In this way, abnormalities can be identified despite their absence on plain films (Figures 2.9, 2.10).[21] Bone scintigraphy is a very sensitive imaging study, however it is of low specificity. Bone scans are valuable in diagnosing infectious discitis or the presence of metastatic disease,[23] and should be considered when the history suggests an osseous lesion.[24] Metastatic disease, particularly in a patient without a known primary, may be an unsuspected source of spine pain. A bone scan may be positive months before plain films will show destructive lesions.[25]

Bone scans can determine if a pars defect is active, providing a dynamic interpretation to a plain film finding. When spondylolysis is seen on X-ray following a work injury, a normal bone scan may provide objective documentation that this is a preexisting finding. Bone scans may remain positive for months and sometimes for over a year after an acute injury.[18] Furthermore, the use of Single Photon Emission Computed Tomography (SPECT) bone scintigraphy improves the clarity of the image resulting in diagnostic advantages,[19] especially when looking at the posterior elements.[20]

Since positive bone scans can help localize the source of a patient's pain, they should be part of a multimodal approach to the evaluation of back pain.[22] In sacroiliitis, SPECT scanning was more specific but not more sensitive than MRI. Therefore, if a SPECT scan was negative but the condition was still suspected, an MRI would be helpful.[26] The bone scan can help direct thin slice CT evaluation of this area.

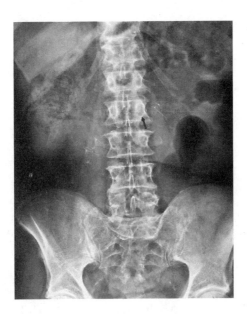

Figure 2.9 Subtle abnormality of left L2 pedicle on X-rays (arrow). With permission.

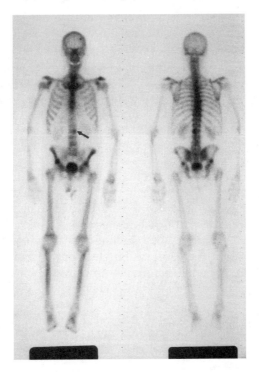

Figure 2.10 Bone scan showing uptake at left L2 pedicle: The patient had metastatic disease.

2.5   Computerized Tomography

Computerized tomography (CT) is a cross-sectional image reconstructed from plain films taken at a variety of preset angles around the central axis of the body. Helical CT scanning provides multiplanar and 3-D reconstruction if clinically indicated. CT gives an excellent view of bone and a better impression of soft tissues than plain films. Conditions such as spurring associated with disc herniation, fracture, spinal stenosis, osteomyelitis, tumor, and facet arthrosis are imaged well with CT (Figures 2.11–2.13). Intrathecal abnormalities are typically poorly defined with CT.

The use of CT has largely been replaced by MRI. There is data however that has shown CT to be comparable to MRI in the diagnosis of disc herniation.[27] CT was found to be an adequate preoperative test in a Finnish study, but this report also showed that the vast majority of patients (86%) evaluated did not have surgery.[28] CT may be the test of choice to study the degeneration of the posterior vertebral structures,[29] but like most imaging studies, it alone cannot determine if the facet arthrosis seen is the pain generator.[30] CT does have a high false positive rate, with a 35% rate of abnormalities in asymptomatic patients, 20% of which were read as having a disc herniation.[31] This emphasizes the need to correlate imaging findings with a detailed clinical evaluation.

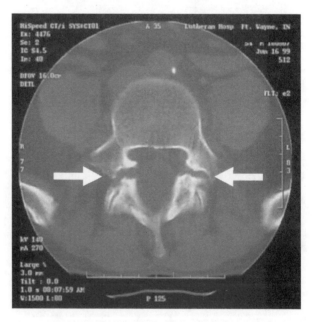

Figure 2.11   CT scan showing bilateral pars interarticularis fractures (arrows).

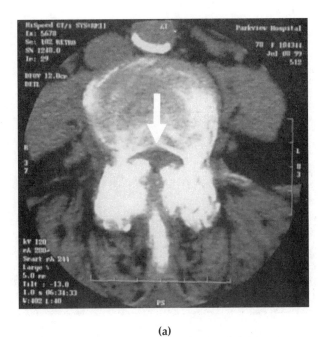

(a)

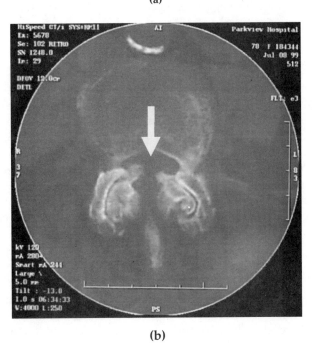

(b)

Figure 2.12a, b CT scan showing advanced spinal stenosis (arrows) on both soft tissue windows (a) and bone windows (b).

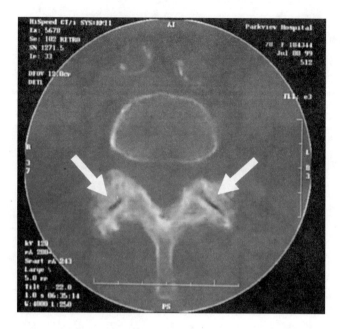

Figure 2.13   CT scan showing advanced facet joint arthrosis (arrows).

2.6 *Myelography*

Myelography involves the injection of contrast material into the dural sac (Figure 2.14). Extradural and intrathecal masses may then be seen involving the contrast material column. Myelography is an invasive test and can commonly cause spinal fluid leaks. Also, as is the case with other spinal imaging tests, false-positive and false-negative findings are not uncommon. Myelography is rarely used as the sole test. A CT scan is often used with myelography to define the diameter of the spinal canal and the effect of any external compression on the canal. Both images are effective individually[1] and together they are complementary,[32] with reported improvement of CT findings by up to 30% with the addition of myelography.[18]

2.7 *Magnetic Resonance Imaging*

Magnetic resonance imaging (MRI) is performed using a strong magnetic field which directs atomic nuclei to align along the directions of the field. This field is bombarded with short pulses of radio waves with the nuclei absorbing energy. As the radiofrequency source is removed, the nuclei release energy which is recorded. The relaxation to the nonexcited state, proton density, and radiofrequency are all determinants of the image generated. The use of MRI has several advantages that have led to its popularity. The study is non-

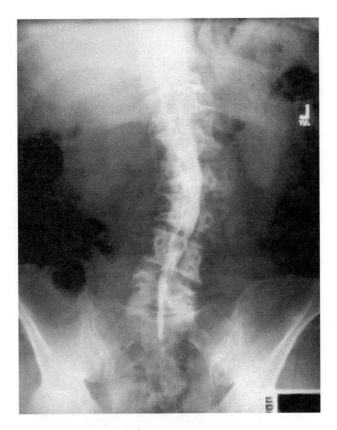

Figure 2.14 Myelogram in patient with scoliosis.

invasive and there is no exposure to ionizing radiation. The entire lumbosacral spine can be included in the imaging field, with the capacity to evaluate multiple planes, most commonly sagittal and axial.

Limitations of the study include claustrophobia, although this has improved with larger scanners and open magnets. Patients with pacemakers or metal implants are typically unable to undergo MRI. When compared to CT, the cost of MRI is usually much higher and therefore is to be considered. In a study by Liu and Byrne, eliminating MRIs ordered outside of established clinical criteria would have decreased costs by eliminating MRIs in five patients that did not meet the diagnostic criteria out of 14 tests that were done. However, there were eight patients that met the criteria but did not get an MRI. Following the criteria precisely would have increased the total costs.[11]

MRI is the most accurate and sensitive modality for diagnosis of subtle occult changes in low back pain.[21] MRI has been recommended as the procedure of choice in evaluating lumbar pathology, replacing CT and myelography.[33] Not only can MRI evaluate the size of the spinal canal, it can also determine what is compromising the canal.[2] MRI is equal in accuracy to plain CT in diagnosing nerve compression due to disc pathology[21, 27] and superior in imaging the cauda equina, the conus medularis, disc degeneration, marrow metastatic disease, inflammatory and neoplastic disease involving the soft tissues, and stenosis (Figures 2.15, 2.16).[23, 29, 34, 35] MRI has the capacity to delineate tears in the annulus that would normally be missed with any other test. MRI may be able to discern between acute symptomatic changes in the disc, which can be associated with hypermobility of the lumbar segment, and generally asymptomatic degenerative changes.[36]

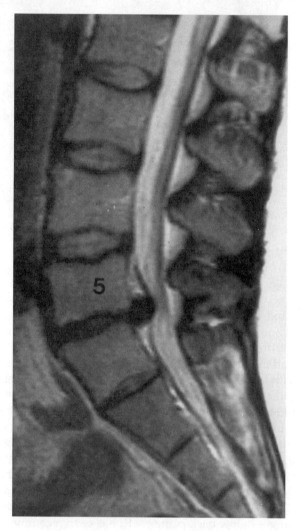

Figure 2.15   MRI sagittal view showing large L5-S1 disc herniation (arrow). With permission.

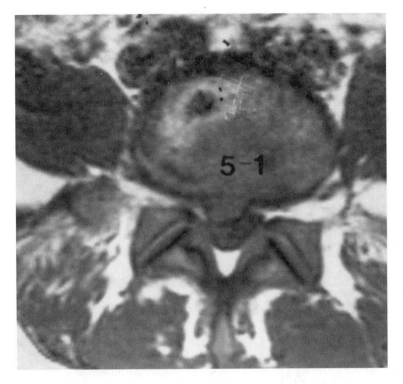

Figure 2.16 MRI axial view showing large L5-S1 disc herniation (arrow).

MRI is not recommended in the first four weeks of low back pain unless specific indications are present. Emergent MRI is warranted in the setting of cauda equina syndrome and rapidly progressing weakness. It may also be helpful in the acute phase to identify suspected tumor, infection, or fracture.[15]

MRI is very sensitive and has a high false positive rate. Twenty to 60% of asymptomatic individuals have an abnormality on MRI.[25, 37, 38] Disc bulging was noted by Jensen in 52% of asymptomatic patients, with 27% shown to have disc protrusions.[37] Considering these studies, the use of all imaging tests should be a part of a comprehensive evaluation, with results considered based upon all available clinical evidence.

2.8 Discography

Discography is a provocative test that determines if a particular interverte-bral disc is the pain generator for an individual with back pain. It is done by injecting a contrast material into the substance of the disc (Figure 2.17). It is controversial in that the test is operator-dependent. Provocation of pain makes discography a functional test, more than an imaging study. In this way

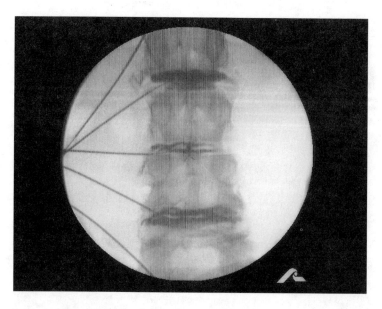

Figure 2.17 Lumbar discography with needles in place and contrast injected at multiple levels.

it can help the primary physician and the surgeon identify if the disc is the pain generator.[39] Bernard reported that the discs were normal in all aspects of imaging, but the discography procedure reproduced the patient's pain. Normal patients as controls were not included. Antti-Poika, et al., found discography helpful to assess discogenic pain in patients who had already undergone posterior fusion. These patients subsequently underwent anterior fusion. They did not feel that postdiscography CT scan added much information and felt that the procedure was worthwhile if MRI was not available.[40] Schneiderman, et al., did not feel that discography was indicated in the setting of a normal MRI.[41]

2.9   Thermography

Thermography is purported to be a picture of pain and a noninvasive means of diagnosing radiculopathies.[42] It measures skin temperature and may be helpful in monitoring the effect of sympathetic nerve blocks in regional pain disorders. However, in an analysis of the available literature, thermography did not localize specific nerve root entrapment or determine the source of nerve root irritation. It is not felt to be of significant benefit in the diagnosis of low back pain.[43] A 1991 meta-analysis of 28 studies out of 81 citations found that only one study was of reasonably high quality and this study did not find any discriminant value in thermography.[44]

2.10 Summary

When choosing a specific diagnostic study, the history and physical exam, the probable diagnosis, and the disorders natural history should be considered in order to minimize the likelihood of imaging study overutilization. Unless "red flags" are present, imaging studies are not recommended within the first four weeks of injury.

Caring for the injured worker with low back pain presents the physician with significant challenges. When ordered appropriately, imaging studies can provide essential information, which impacts directly on treatment decision making. However, many of these tests are expensive and have been reported to have many false positives. Therefore, an imaging study should be ordered when the results will impact subsequent treatment plans.

2.11 References

1. Bosacco, S. J., Berman, A. T., Garbarino, J. L. et al. A comparison of CT scanning and myelography in the diagnosis of lumbar disc herniation, *Clin. Orthop. & Related Res.* 190:124, 1984.
2. Boos, N., Lander Ph. H. Clinical efficacy of imaging modalities in the diagnosis of low-back pain disorders, *Eur. Spine* 1, 5, 2, 1996.
3. Boden, L. I. Worker's compensation in the United States: High costs, low benefits. *Annu. Rev. Public Health,* 16:189, 1995.
4. Baker, L. C., Krueger, A. B. Medical costs in worker's compensation insurance, *J. of Health Econ.* 14:531, 1995.
5. Johnson, W. C., Baldwin, M. L., Burton, J. F., Jr. Why is the treatment of work-related injuries so costly? New evidence from California, *Inquiry* 33:53, 1996.
6. Johnson, W. C., Butler, R., Baldwin, M. et al. The cost-effectiveness of alternative treatments for low back pain abstract. *AHSR & FHSR Annual Meeting Abstract Book,* 11:138.
7. Swedlow, A., Johnson, C., Smithline, N. et al. Increased costs and rates of use in the California worker's compensation system as a result of self-referral by physicians, *N. Eng. J. Med.,* 327:1502, 1992.
8. Carey, T. S., Garrett, J. The North Carolina Back Pain Project. Patterns of ordering diagnostic tests for patients with acute low back pain, *Ann. Intern. Med.* 125:807, 1996.
9. Elam, K. C., Cherkin, D. C, Deyo, R. A. How emergency physicians approach low back pain: Choosing costly options. *J. Emerg. Med.* 13:143, 1995.
10. Schroth, W. S., Schectman, J. M., Elinsky, E. C. et al. Utilization of medical services of the treatment of low back pain: Conformance with clinical guidelines, *J. Gen. Intern. Med.,* 7:486, 1992.
11. Liu, A. C., Byrne, E. Cost of care for ambulatory patients with low back pain, *J. of Family Practice,* 40:449, 1995.
12. Wise, D. How providing more care costs less, *Business & Health,* 12:67, 1994.
13. Chakera, T. M. H., McCormick, C. C. Radiology and low back pain. *Aust. Fam. Physician,* 24:1995.

14. Scavone, J. C., Latshaw, R. F., Rohrar GV. Use of lumbar spine films: Statistical evaluation at a university teaching hospital. *JAMA* 246:1105–1108, 1981.
15. Agency For Health Care Policy and Research, U.S. Department of Health and Human Services. Acute low back pain in adults, December, 1994.
16. Deyo, R. A. Early diagnostic evaluation of low back pain. *J. Gen. Intern. Med.*, 1:328, 1986.
17. Rhea, J. T., DeLuca, S. A., et al. The oblique view: An unnecessary component of the adult lumbar spine examination. *Radiology* 134:45–47, 1980.
18. Boden, S. D. Diagnostic imaging of the spine. *Essentials of the Spine.* (New York: Raven Press, 1995) 97–110.
19. Howarth, D., Southee, A., Cardew, F. et al. SPECT in avulsion injury of the multifidus and rotator muscles of the lumbar region, *Clin. Nucl. Med.*, 19:571, 1994.
20. Ryan, P. J., Evans, P. A., Gibson, T. et al. Chronic low back pain: Comparison of bone SPECT with radiography and CT, *Radiology*, 182:849, 1992.
21. Sluming, V. A., Scutt, N. D. The role of imaging in the diagnosis of postural disorders related to low back pain, *Sports Med.* 18:281, 1994.
22. Collier, B. D., Kir, K. M., Mills, B. J. A. et al. Bone scan: A useful test for evaluating patients with low back pain, *Skeletal Radiol.* 19:267, 1990.
23. Luers, P. R. Lumbosacral spine imaging: Physioanatomic method, *Curr. Probl. Diagn. Radiol.* 21:151, 1992.
24. Ryan, R. J., Gibson, T., Fogelman, I. The identification of spinal pathology in chronic low back pain using single photon emission computed tomography, *Nucl. Med. Commun.* 13:497, 1992.
25. Al-Janabi, M. A. Imaging modalities and low back pain: The role of bone scintigraphy, *Nucl. Med. Commun.* 16:317, 1995.
26. Hanly, J. G., Mitchell, M. J., Barnes, D. C. et al. Early recognition of sacroiliitis by magnetic resonance imaging and single photon emission computed tomography, *Rheumatology,* 21:2088, 1994.
27. Thornbury, J. R., Fryback, D. G., Turski, P. A., et al. Disc-caused nerve compression in patients with acute low back pain: Diagnosis with MRI, CT myelography, and plain CT. *Radiology* 186:731–738, 1992.
28. Ilkko, E., Lahde, S. Computed tomography as the primary radiological examination of lumbar spine, *Roentgen-Blatter,* 41:414, 1988.
29. Monti, C., Busacca, M., Bettini, N. et al. Modern diagnostic imaging of lumbar spondylosis, *Chirurgia Degli Organi di Movimento,* 79:19, 1994.
30. Schwarzer, A. C., Shih-Chang, W., O'Driscoll, D. et al. The ability of computed tomography to identify a painful zygapophysial joint in patients with chronic low back pain, *Spine,* 20:907, 199.
31. Wiesel, S. W., Tsourmas, N., Feffer, H. L. et al. A study of computer assisted tomography. 1. The incidence of positive CT scans in an asymptomatic group of patients. *Spine* 9:549–551, 1984.
32. Witt, I., Vestergaard, A., Rosenklint, A. A comparative analysis of x-ray findings of the lumbar spine in patients with and without pain. *Spine* 9:298–300, 1984.
33. Takahashi, M. et al. Comparison of magnetic resonance imaging with myelography and computed tomography-myelography in the diagnosis of lumbar disc herniation. *Neuroimaging Clin. of N. Amer.* August, 1993 3(3):487–498.
34. Herzog, R. J., Guyer, R. D., Graham-Smith, A. et al. Magnetic resonance imaging use in patients with low back or radicular pain, *Spine,* 20, 1834, 1995.

35. Jensen, M. C., Kelly, A. P., Brant-Zawadzki, M. N. MRI of degenerative disease of the lumbar spine, *Mag. Resonance Q.* 10:173, 1994.
36. Toyone, T., Takahashi, K., Kitahara, H. et al. Vertebral bone marrow changes in degenerative lumbar disc disease, *J. Bone and J. Surg. (Br.)*, 76-B:757, 1994.
37. Jensen, M. C., Brant-Zawadki, M. N., Obuchowski, N. et al. Magnetic resonance imaging of the lumbar spine in people without back pain. *JAMA*, 331:69, 1994.
38. Wiesel, S. The reliability of imaging (computed tomography, magnetic resonance imaging, myelography) in documenting the cause of spinal pain. *J. Manipulative & Physiol. Ther.* 15:51, 1992.
39. Bernard, T. N. Lumbar discography followed by computed tomography. Refining the diagnosis of low-back pain, *Spine*, 15:690, 1990.
40. Antti-Poika, I., Soini, J., Tallroth, K. et al. Clinical relevance of discography combined with CT scanning, *JBJS (Br.)* 72-B:480, 1990.
41. Schneiderman, G., Flannigan, B., Kingston, S. et al. Magnetic resonance imaging in the diagnosis of disc degeneration: Correlation with discography, *Spine*, 12:276, 1987.
42. Thomas, D. Infrared thermographic imaging, magnetic resonance imaging, CT scan and myelography in low back pain. *Br. J. of Rheumatol.* 29:268, 1990.
43. Pawl, R. Thermography in the diagnosis of low back pain, *Neurosurg. Clin. of N. Amer.* 2:839, 1991.
44. Hoffman, R. M., Kent, D. L., Deyo, R. A. Diagnostic accuracy and clinical utility of thermography for lumbar radiculopathy: A metanalysis. *Spine*, 16:623, 1991.

chapter three

Electrodiagnosis and Lumbar Spine Disorders

Mayra I. Alfonso, M.D.
Bryan D. Kaplansky, M.D.
Jacqueline J. Wertsch, M.D.

3.1 Overview

3.1.1 What is electrodiagnostic medicine?

The beginnings of electromyography might be traced to Adrian and Bronk who recorded muscle activity with a concentric needle electrode in 1929.[2] Many people use the general term EMG when they refer to electrodiagnostic studies. In fact, the electrodiagnostic medicine consultation uses two different types of neurophysiologic data: NCS (nerve conduction studies) and needle EMG (electromyography).

Nerve conduction studies are, as the name implies, a study of conduction in a nerve. To do this, a nerve is stimulated and the resultant response is recorded. If the response is recorded from a sensory nerve, is called a sensory nerve action potential (SNAP). If the response is recorded from a muscle, information about the motor nerves is provided and the response is called a compound muscle action potential (CMAP).

With needle EMG there is no stimulation. Instead a needle is inserted into a muscle and the electrical activity generated by the muscle fibers is recorded. This electrode can detect changes in the electrical stability of the muscle membrane (caused by neuropathic, myopathic, or metabolic processes) and can also be used to examine the electrical properties of the muscle during voluntary contraction.

0-8493-0089-4/00/$0.00+$.50
© 2000 by CRC Press LLC

Since NCS and needle EMG are two very different procedures, the term electrodiagnostic study is the preferred term. In some instances, both needle EMG and NCS are required to evaluate a patient's condition; in other instances, only needle EMG or only NCS will be necessary. Which study to perform is determined by the electrodiagnostic consultant and will depend on the question being asked by the referring physician and on the differential diagnosis.

A frequently asked question is: What is the appropriate test a referring physician should order to evaluate a patient for a specific clinical condition, EMG or NCS? The referring physician should specify what is the question which he wants the electromyographer to answer, letting the consulted electromyographer decide what is the best electrodiagnostic (EDx) approach to evaluate the patient condition. For example, the patient referral could say "EDx to rule out left lumbosacral radiculopathy" or "EDx to rule out left carpal tunnel syndrome." There is no need to specify if needle EMG or nerve conduction studies should be performed.

Electrodiagnostic testing evaluates the physiologic integrity of the peripheral nervous system. It is very different from radiologic studies, such as X-rays, CT scans, or MRI scans. Comparing radiologic studies and electrodiagnostic studies is somewhat like comparing apples and oranges. Radiologic studies assess anatomy whereas electrodiagnostic testing assesses physiology. Electrodiagnostic testing is a valuable tool in the assessment of peripheral polyneuropathies, radiculopathies, myopathies, motor neuron diseases, and focal peripheral nerve entrapments such as peroneal neuropathies.

A patient saying, "I had an EMG, and it was negative" is similar to a patient saying, "I had blood work done, and it was negative." Without further details about what was actually done, either statement is not very helpful. Electrodiagnostic testing is really an extension of the history and physical examination. It is another tool for gathering physiologic information during the physical examination, analogous in this sense to the use of a reflex hammer. Therefore, electrodiagnostic testing is part of a consultation and not merely a "lab test." As a consultation, electrodiagnostic testing can be ordered early in a workup to help establish or narrow the differential diagnosis, or it can be requested later to help confirm a clinical diagnosis. In either scenario, EDx testing accomplishes its goals by evaluating the physiologic status of the various components of the peripheral nervous system. A carefully planned, well-directed study can help diagnose disorders of any part of the peripheral nervous system, including the sensory nerve fibers and the motor unit (anterior horn cell, nerve root, cervical or lumbosacral plexus, peripheral nerves, neuromuscular junction, and muscle).

When the electromyographer evaluates a patient he or she should perform a focused history and physical examination, which is followed by the EDx study. Therefore, the EDx testing should be an extension of a history and physical exam and it should be performed as a consultation by the electromyographer. The EDx testing should be carefully planned, taking into account the patient's history and physical examination, and should be modified depending on the findings encountered during the study.

The findings on EDx testing should be internally consistent with the patient's history and physical examination. For example, the needle EMG exam abnormalities for a patient with a right L4 lumbosacral radiculopathy, should be detected only in the L4 root innervated muscles of the right lower limb. If no such abnormalities are detected, or if abnormalities are observed in other than L4 root innervated muscles, the diagnosis of L4 lumbosacral radiculopathy should be reconsidered.

3.1.2 Who should perform the electrodiagnostic studies?

There is marked variation in the training received by physicians who perform electrodiagnostic testing. Currently, any physician can attend a weekend technical instructional course given by a machine manufacturer, buy a machine, and legally perform electrodiagnostic studies. The only American specialty board that requires training in electrodiagnostic medicine during residency is Physical Medicine and Rehabilitation (PM&R). To become board-eligible in PM&R, a resident must have "a minimum of three months" of training in electromyography. One-year fellowships in electrodiagnostic medicine are available. Currently there is no credentialing mechanism for EMG fellowships, so the content and focus can vary tremendously from one program to another. Also, there is no list of physicians who have completed EMG fellowships; thus, without asking directly, the referring physician has no way of knowing whether an electromyographer completed a fellowship.

The American Association of Electromyography and Electrodiagnosis (AAEE) was founded in 1953. The purpose of the organization was "to maximize understanding of neuromuscular disorders though appropriate use of clinical electromyography and related neurophysiologic techniques by promoting programs of education, research, and quality assurance." The AAEE began to give a voluntary examination in 1967. Although the AAEE examination evolved from the educational mission of the organization, the examination was increasingly viewed as a certification of competency in the field of clinical neurophysiology. In 1987, the AAEE approved the concept of separating its membership and examination functions. Thus, a completely autonomous, independent certifying board was established—the American Board of Electrodiagnostic Medicine (ABEM). The AAEE continues as a purely educational organization under the name of the American Association of Electrodiagnostic Medicine (AAEM). The ABEM gave its first examination in April, 1989. A directory of ABEM Diplomates is readily available from the ABEM offices:

American Board of Electrodiagnostic Medicine (ABEM)
21 Second Street S.W., Suite 306
Rochester, MN 55902
Telephone: (507) 288–0100
Fax: (507) 288–1225

3.2 Pathophysiology of Neuronal Injury

3.2.1 Types of Injuries

Two types of nerve injuries occur: injury to the myelin or injury to the axons. There are multiple etiologies for nerve injuries: laceration of the nerve, stretching of the nerve, compression by external pressure, ischemia, radiation, or infiltration of malignant cells. Nerve injuries are not only classified by their etiology, but they are also classified by their pathophysiology. Seddon introduced the terms neurapraxia, axonotmesis, and neurotmesis to classify the neuronal injuries (Table 3.1).[25] It is important to identify what kind of pathophysiology is involved with neuronal injury, since this will help determine the patient's prognosis. The best prognosis is when both the myelin and axon are physically intact and there is simply a focal conduction block.

Neurapraxia is defined as a temporary conduction block. It is usually caused by entrapment of the nerve, without loss of architectural structure. In neurapraxia, the myelin sheath that surrounds the nerve is affected, without disrupting the axons. When the myelin is affected, the saltatory conduction of the nerve impulse becomes abnormal, producing an expected slowing of conduction in the involved segment. A normal nerve conduction velocity with a normal latency and amplitude of the action potential is observed distal to the area of neurapraxia.

Neurapraxia is the mildest form of conduction block. It may last for minutes, hours, days, or longer, and it is usually reversible. It can resolve after a nerve entrapment is released. An example of neurapraxia is the use of local anesthetics that block the nerve transmission. Another example of neurapraxia occurs when a person crosses his/her legs while sitting and develops transient paresthesias down the limb. If the external pressure on the nerve persists for prolonged periods of time or involves a big area, structural changes within the nerve will start to occur and the term neurapraxia will no longer apply. In this case the term axonotmesis would be more appropriate.

Axonotmesis is considered a moderate form of nerve damage, in which interruption of the physical integrity of the axon occurs. The endoneurium, perineurium and epineurium, (which are the connective tissues that surround the individual nerve axons), and the nerve fascicles are preserved. Due to axonal damage, signs of denervation will appear on needle EMG studies. NCS in this situation will not only show a prolonged latency in sensory

Table 3.1 Types of Nerve Injury

Neurapraxia: Conduction block due to involvement of myelin sheath: slowing of nerve conduction for the involved segment on NCS. Normal conduction proximal and distal to lesion.

Axonotmesis: Axonal damage: prolonged latency and low amplitude of action potential on NCS; denervation and abnormal MUAPs on EMG.

Neurotmesis: Complete interruption of axon and connective tissue: no action potential on NCS; denervation and no MUAPs on EMG.

and/or motor studies due to demyelination, but also will show evidence of low amplitudes due to axonal loss.

Neurotmesis is the most severe form of nerve damage. A complete interruption of the nerve, including the axons and their connective tissue is observed. No nerve conduction is able to be obtained across the site of injury. On needle EMG, there is evidence of complete denervation. An example of neurotmesis is nerve transection secondary to a traumatic injury such as a laceration or a severe traction injury. NCS would reveal a complete absence of responses and marked denervation abnormalities would be noted on needle EMG with no motor unit action potentials (MUAPs) present.

3.2.2   Chronology of Abnormalities

There is a known sequence of electrodiagnostic abnormalities which follows a fairly predictable time course following a nerve injury (Table 3.4).[1, 3, 4, 12, 14, 22] The details of what happens when depends on what type of injury there was and the site of the injury. Immediately after a complete lesion (neurotmesis), needle EMG examination shows no MUAPs in the muscles distal to the injury site, and nerve conduction studies across the site of a complete lesion demonstrate no detectable response. In contrast, the nerve distal to the complete lesion remains temporarily functional, and conduction studies performed with both the stimulus site and the recording site distal to the injury location will be normal for approximately two to three days, except for the absence of detectable H-reflex and F-wave responses. At about that time, the CMAP amplitude begins to decrease until it is no longer detectable at about seven to nine days. The SNAP amplitude begins to decrease at about five days and becomes undetectable at about 10 days.

How soon abnormalities appear on the needle EMG examination depends on the distance between the nerve lesion and the muscle fibers innervated by the injured axons. Since Wallerian degeneration proceeds from proximal to distal, the more proximal muscles will show evidence of denervation first. For example, following axonal damage to a nerve root, evidence of muscle membrane instability is seen in the paraspinal muscles by about Day 7, in the proximal limb muscles by about Day 14, and in the distal limb muscles by about Day 21.[12] Additionally, if a nerve injury is incomplete (axonotmesis), the needle EMG examination may reveal MUAP recruitment abnormalities. Thus, there are many known physiologic phenomena with recognized time courses that affect the findings on electrodiagnostic examination.

3.3   Electrodiagnostic Studies

There are several types of electrodiagnostic studies that are utilized to evaluate low back and lower limb disorders (Table 3.2). In NCS, a small electrical current is applied to the nerve, producing a wave form. In needle EMG, a small needle electrode is inserted into the muscle and the electrical activity

Table 3.2   Electrodiagnostic Studies

1. Needle electromyography.
   a. Routine needle electromyography (EMG).
   b. Single fiber electromyography (SFEMG).
2. Nerve conduction studies.
   a. Sensory nerve conduction studies (SNCS).
   b. Motor nerve conduction studies (MNCS).
   c. Late responses—H reflex and F wave.
   d. Somatosensory evoked potentials (SSEP).

produced is observed. Needle EMG is most commonly used in the evaluation of a lumbosacral radiculopathy.

3.3.1   Needle Electromyography

To rule out a possible lumbosacral radiculopathy, for evaluation of a patient with low back pain, needle EMG is usually performed on the affected limb or limbs and on the lumbosacral paraspinal muscles. Which muscles of the lower extremity are examined during an evaluation of a patient to rule out a lumbosacral radiculopathy will vary from one examiner to another. To perform needle EMG of the lower limbs, the patient will lie supine in a comfortable position to permit easy assess to the leg muscles (Figure 3.1). To examine the lumbosacral paraspinal muscles, the patient may lie on one side or prone.

The needle electrode that is inserted in the muscle can detect changes in the electrical stability of the muscle cell membrane and also can examine the electrical properties of the muscle during contraction. A normal muscle cell is electrically silent at rest. The normal transmembrane potential is not detected

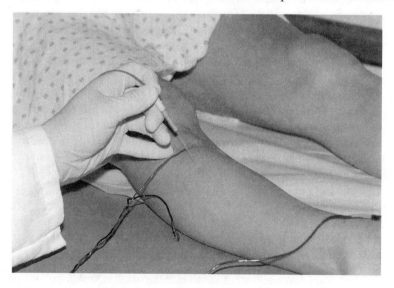

Figure 3.1   Needle electromyography.

by the needle EMG examination because the needle tip remains outside of the muscle cell membrane. In denervation, the muscle cell will be more irritable than normal and can even spontaneously depolarize. The needle EMG study can detect this increased muscle membrane irritability during insertional activity. Insertional activity is defined as the burst of potentials produced immediately after inserting a needle electrode into a resting muscle. This activity should cease immediately after the needle stops moving. Insertional activity might be abnormally prolonged, persisting beyond the time during which the needle is inserted, if the muscle membrane has increased irritability. Prolonged insertional activity is a nonspecific finding and can be observed in denervation or in myopathic processes. Insertional activity can be decreased or totally absent in atrophied muscles.

With denervation, the resting muscle cell no longer remains electrically silent but will spontaneously depolarize and produce "spontaneous potentials." The spontaneous potentials can take several different shapes. The most commonly encountered in lumbosacral radiculopathies are positive waves and fibrillation potentials which are collectively referred to as "spontaneous single muscle fiber discharges" or SSFDs. The size of the positive sharp waves and fibrillation potentials can help identify whether a process is acute or chronic. During an acute process the denervation potentials are being produced by large muscle cells so the potentials are large (perhaps 200–800 Vs). In a chronic process where the muscle cells have atrophied, the potentials will be small (perhaps 10–20 Vs).[15] This can be very useful information for the occupational physician who desires to sort out whether a lumbosacral radiculopathy is acute or chronic.

When an anterior horn cell is activated during a voluntary muscle contraction, the wave of depolarization travels down its axon to excite, virtually simultaneously, all the muscle fibers supplied by that anterior horn cell. Since these muscle fibers discharge at approximately the same instant, they will be summated into a single large waveform, the MUAP. The amplitude and shape (or morphology) of the MUAP are determined by the number and synchrony of the muscle fibers that are recorded. In lumbosacral radiculopathy, if the conduction to some muscle fibers is compromised, the synchrony of the muscle fiber contractions will be affected and the MUAP can appear polyphasic and have a low amplitude. In contrast, if a motor axon has reinnervated previously denervated muscle fibers belonging to a neighboring motor unit, then the added muscle fibers augment the MUAP amplitude. The resultant MUAP will be large and polyphasic. MUAP analysis is playing an increasingly important part in the EMG exam and should be included in every study.

3.3.2 Nerve Conduction Studies

Nerve conduction studies are useful in diagnosing focal peripheral neuropathies such as peroneal nerve entrapment in the lower extremity. Also, NCS are useful in the diagnosis of peripheral polyneuropathy which can result from diabetes mellitus, alcohol use and many other etiologies. It is not extremely useful in the diagnosis of lumbosacral radiculopathies; however, a preserved SNAP can demonstrate the preganglionic site of root entrapment.

In performing NCS, a stimulus is applied over a nerve. This impulse is transmitted from the stimulation site and is recorded at some other site along the nerve. The electromyographer evaluates the speed of transmission from the stimulation site to the recording site and records the latency and conduction velocity. It is also important to note the amplitude and duration of the action potential generated by the applied stimulus.

NCS are divided into motor nerve conduction studies (MNCS) and sensory nerve conduction studies (SNCS). The MNCS response is recorded from a muscle innervated by the stimulated nerve and is known as the compound motor action potential (CMAP) (Figure 3.2). The SNCS response is recorded from the sensory nerve itself and is known as the sensory nerve action potential (SNAP) (Figure 3.3).

When onset latencies are used, the latency is determined by the speed of conduction of the fastest motor axons, the large myelinated motor fibers.

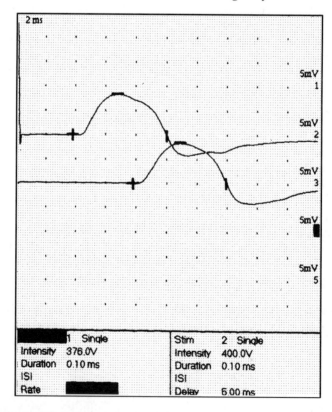

Figure 3.2   Compound motor action potential.

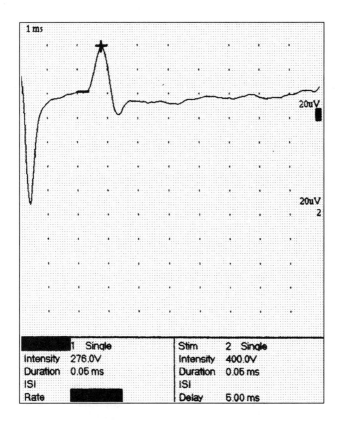

Figure 3.3 Sensory nerve action potential.

These fibers are more sensitive to injury, and are selectively affected with gradual compression. Peak latencies are also utilized by electromyographers. To calculate conduction velocity, two sites on the nerve are stimulated and the latency difference is divided into the length of nerve segment between the two stimulation sites. A typical nerve conduction velocity is 50 meters/second in the arms and 40 meters/second in the legs. Thus, nerves are normally conducting at speeds of about 100 miles per hour.

In the lower extremities, the most frequent motor nerves studied are the tibial and peroneal nerves and the most frequent sensory nerves studied are the sural and superficial peroneal nerves. Motor and sensory nerve conduction studies are often normal in radiculopathies. The SNAP is commonly preserved in radiculopathies because the site of root compromise is usually proximal to the dorsal root ganglia. In MNCS, the amplitude of the CMAP could be abnormally low if the radiculopathy is causing axonal loss. For example, a L5 or S1 radiculopathy may cause a low amplitude in the peroneal or tibial nerve CMAPs.

3.3.3   Late Responses H Reflex and F Wave

H reflexes and F waves are called late responses because they appear "late" after the CMAP in MNCS. The F waves are called "F" because they were initially recorded from the foot muscles. They were first described by Magladery and McDougal in 1950.[19] Every time the motor nerve is stimulated, the wave of depolarization spreads both proximally and distally from the site of stimulation. The wave traveling proximally toward the spinal cord can "rebound" off the anterior horn cell. It will then travel back down the nerve past the original site of stimulation to the muscle where it is recorded as a small muscle response.[19, 2, 5, 6, 8, 20, 21] The F-wave potential is small because "rebound" occurs in only about 1–5% of the stimulated motor axons.[2, 7, 18, 24] F waves are variable; therefore, repeated stimulation produces F waves of different latencies and wave form morphology. This is due to the fact that different motor axons are stimulated each time. A minimum of eight to ten responses are usually done during F-wave testing.

The F wave latencies represent conduction through the whole length of the motor nerve. Therefore, they are useful in evaluating proximal nerve lesions such as plexopathies or radiculopathies. They also can be important in identifying Guillain-Barré syndrome or multifocal demyelinating processes. If only the sensory axons are damaged, the F wave will remain normal, because it only depends on the motor axons' integrity. Other parameters used in the evaluation of F waves are their size, dispersion of the waveform, and persistency in which it appears. Abnormal persistence of F waves may be a clue to investigate for a possible focal neuropathy due to impingement from a central disk herniation.[27]

A few limitations of F waves are known. F wave studies may be normal in lumbosacral radiculopathies. When abnormal, they may not add much information to a needle EMG study in which evidence of radiculopathy had been found.[28] They only assess the integrity of motor fibers; therefore, if only the sensory fibers are affected, they are not useful. An isolated abnormal F wave is not diagnostic of radiculopathy and F waves do not localize the lesion to the root level. Also, abnormal F waves do not distinguish radiculopathies from plexopathies. They can be critically important, however, to alerting the clinician to proximal demyelinating processes that may present clinically like a radiculopathy.

The H reflex is defined as a monosynaptic spinal reflex. It is bigger than the F wave, almost as big as the CMAP. It was first described by Hoffman in 1918, and it is named after him.[2] In newborns the H reflex can be elicited in almost every muscle. In adults only in a few muscles can the H reflex be elicited. In adults the most commonly studied is the soleus H reflex. The tibial nerve is stimulated in the popliteal fossa with the response recorded from the soleus muscle in the calf.

The H reflex is felt by some to be useful for assessing the S1 root. Some limitations to the H reflex are known. The H reflex can become abnormal with the onset of root compression and remain abnormal even after the compression has ceased. Thus it offers little assistance in evaluating patients with history of prior S1 radiculopathy. The H reflex is mediated over a long pathway, including the sciatic and tibial nerves, sacral plexus, spinal cord, and S1 motor and sensory roots;[28] therefore, lesions at any of these levels can cause identical H wave abnormalities as seen in S1 radiculopathy. Therefore, the H reflex study has a low specificity. A finding of an abnormal H wave is not diagnostic of an S1 radiculopathy, because H waves are frequently not obtained bilaterally in patients with peripheral polyneuropathies and in normal subjects over 60 years of age.[28] They are also usually absent bilaterally following a lumbar laminectomy, even when the surgery was on the contralateral side.

3.3.4 Somatosensory-Evoked Potentials

Somatosensory-evoked potentials (SSEP) are similar to nerve conduction studies in that a nerve is stimulated, and a response is recorded. The difference is that the response is recorded from the spinal cord and brain. Mixed nerves are commonly stimulated, although some like to stimulate cutaneous nerves. Dermatomal stimulation has also been reported. The most commonly stimulated nerves are the posterior tibial and peroneal nerves.

In SSEP, the latency of the individual responses and the interval between different responses are examined and correlated to height. The amplitude and the presence or absence of individual responses are also studied. It is out of the scope of this chapter to review all the technical aspects involved in SSEP testing. Additional specific information is available in an electrodiagnostic text.

SSEP might help in the evaluation of patients with suspected radiculopathy, because they can assess sensory function in proximal portions of the peripheral nervous system. However, SSEP have limitations. Due to the long distance between the site of peripheral stimulation and the central nervous system site where the responses are recorded, a focal slowing of conduction due to compression of nerve fibers traversing a nerve root may be masked. It can also be falsely negative in the presence of compromised and unaffected sensory fibers within the same nerve or root, because the unaffected fibers will permit normal conduction and mask the slower conducting affected fibers. False positives are also possible in view of the very long segment studied and the recording technicalities. At this time, the utility of SSEP for diagnosing lumbar radiculopathy has not been firmly established.

3.3.5 Single-Fiber Electromyography

Single-fiber electromyography (SFEMG) is a specialized technique utilized to study an individual muscle cell.[26] A special needle electrode is put into a muscle and focused on a pair of muscle cells from one motor unit. The variation in latency differences between the two muscle fiber action potentials indicates the "jitter." Fiber density is also recorded by systematically recording from different areas. The technique is time-consuming and requires skill and a lot of practice by the electromyographer. It is most commonly used to aid in the early diagnosis of myasthenia gravis. It is also used clinically to help assess whether reinnervation after nerve compromise is completed or on-going, which might be a useful application in lumbosacral radiculopathy.

3.4   Clinical Applications in Occupational Low Back Pain

3.4.1   Overview

The electrodiagnostic study is a valuable diagnostic tool in the evaluation of workers with low back pain and associated lower limb symptoms. Electrodiagnostic studies should be ordered when neuromuscular dysfunction needs to be confirmed or excluded as a diagnosis. An electromyogram and nerve conduction studies are generally not indicated in individuals with symptoms isolated to the low back only because an associated neurogenic disorder is usually associated with concomitant limb complaints. Certain conditions may cause isolated low back pain that can be detected by paraspinal needle electrodiagnostic studies, such as a dorsal ramus neuropathy or a local paraspinal muscle disorder.[9] However, these are probably unusual conditions, especially in the injured Workers' Compensation population.

There are many clinical advantages associated with electrodiagnostic studies (Table 3.3). An EMG can localize, qualitate, and quantitate neuromuscular conditions. Nerve conduction studies also assist the clinician with prognostication concerning nerve injuries by determining whether a neuropathy is due to neurapraxia, axonotmesis, or neurotmesis. Furthermore, electrodiagnostic studies can determine the chronicity of a condition such as a radiculopathy by determining whether the needle EMG findings are acute or chronic, which may then have medicolegal implications, particularly in the Worker's Compensation setting.

Electrodiagnostic studies can also help in the institution of a treatment program in certain individuals. Electrodiagnostic studies can help localize the symptomatic nerve root abnormality in the setting of multilevel spinal abnormalities seen on imaging studies. This finding can then allow one to order sophisticated treatment options such as regional epidural blocks directed specifically to the level of radiculopathy. Furthermore, an EMG can confirm the presence of a lumbosacral radiculopathy suspected only on history and physical examination despite the presence of negative or inconclusive imaging studies. Another example is a worker with a previous history of lumbar discectomy who has a recurrence of back and leg pain but a "negative" MRI scan with gadolinium that shows only postsurgical scarring but no recurrent disc herniation. An EMG in such a case may confirm an acute radiculopathy. On the other hand, electrodiagnostic studies can rule out underlying nonoccupational sources that may be contributing to an individual

Table 3.3   Specific Examples of Electrodiagnostic Utilities

Localizes conditions (i.e., sciatic neuropathy versus lumbosacral radiculopathy).

Can help to determine the chronicity of the neuromuscular disorder.

Can diagnose neuromuscular conditions not isolated on imaging studies (i.e., a false-negative MRI or noncompressive radiculitis) and can localize the specific nerve root level in an individual with a radiculopathy and complicated imaging studies (i.e., multilevel problems such as multilevel lumbar spinal stenosis, multilevel disc herniations).

Can help to direct a treatment plan (i.e., an EMG that localizes an L3 radiculopathy that may have not previously responded to medications, physical therapy, and standard lumbar epidural blocks but may respond to an L3 fluoroscopically guided regional epidural block in conjunction with a comprehensive rehabilitation program).

Helpful in postsurgical cases where a recurrent disc may not be noted and only scarring is noted on the MRI but the patient does have an ongoing radiculopathy.

Can rule out underlying concomitant abnormalities (i.e., nonoccupational factors such as a polyneuropathy from diabetes mellitus).

Can assist in prognostication (i.e., axonotmesis versus neurapraxia).

---

worker's complaints such as a peripheral polyneuropathy from diabetes mellitus. It can also rule out other conditions that may mimic radiculopathy such as a peroneal neuropathy at the knee.

An EMG is a sensitive dynamic electrophysiologic test with a low incidence of false-positive results. The sensitivity of a paraspinal and extremity needle exam in the investigation of radiculopathy has been reported to be in the range of 94–98%.[17] The paraspinal needle exam in particular has been shown to be a very sensitive test. Some studies have reported that the paraspinal needle exam is more sensitive for radiculopathies than the peripheral exam alone.[10] Due to the highly sensitive nature of electrodiagnostic studies, investigators have suggested that EMG should be the first test of choice and the initial workup for a lumbar radiculopathy.[13] The same authors report that abnormal electrodiagnostic studies appear to correlate better with a demonstrated course of a radiculopathy than CT.[13]

The sensitivity of electrodiagnostic studies is particularly valuable when the history and clinical physical exam findings and imaging studies do not correlate well. Static anatomic tests are known to yield a high rate of false-positive findings.[11] Misinterpreting the significance of radiographic studies which are fraught with a high rate of false-positive and false-negative findings may lead to erroneus therapeutic decisions. A review of the causes of lumbar discectomy failure revealed that the imaging studies of these patients were poorly correlated with the clinical findings.[23] The needle EMG, on the other hand, is important in determining whether the anatomic findings are functionally or clinically relevant. Some authors[16] report that EMG and imaging studies should be used in a complementary manner: EMG indicating function and imaging studies indicating structure.

3.4.2　When to Order Electrodiagnostic Studies

Ideally an electrodiagnostic test should be performed as early as possible in the course of the disease to serve as a baseline for electrophysiologic function at that time. Results can then be compared with subsequent studies to assess the prognosis for recovery or to follow the severity of the process and the resolution of the abnormality. However, in light of the high rate of recovery with low back injuries with radiculopathy, the EMG and nerve conduction studies should usually be delayed for at least three or four weeks after the development of limb symptoms. There are several reasons for this. An EMG follows a temporal pattern and allows for a dynamic evaluation of neurophysiologic function and dysfunction (Table 3.4).

Although nerve conduction study abnormalities and decreased recruitment of MUAPs can be detected initially at the onset of symptoms, other EMG findings take time to develop.

An EMG may not be necessary in the case of an obvious radiculopathy based on the history and physical examination. Although serial electrodiagnostic studies can help follow the temporal pattern of a neuromuscular disorder, including radiculopathy in an injured worker, this is rarely necessary. In the majority of cases, treatment decisions can be based on careful serial histories and physical examinations in the office. An individual who improves subjectively and objectively does not need serial electrodiagnostic studies to confirm what is already known on the history and physical examination. If the patient does not improve or plateaus, the electrodiagnostic studies could be added to assist in the confirmation of a diagnosis and can help to pattern

Table 3.4　Sequence of Electrodiagnostic Abnormalities in Lumbar Radiculopathy

Days from the onset of injury	Electrodiagnostic Abnormalities
0	Reduced Recruitment Reduced Recruitment Interval Abnormal H reflexes & F waves
0–4	Compound motor action potential amplitude reduced
0–7	Positive waves in paraspinal muscles
0–12 to 14	Positive waves in proximal limb muscles; fibrillation potentials in paraspinal muscles
0–18 to 21	Positive waves and fibrillation potentials in paraspinal and limb muscles
0–5 to 6 weeks	Reinnervation changes for motor unit action potentials
Six months to one year	Increased amplitude of reinnervated motor unit action potentials.

Adapted from Ernest W. Johnson, Electrodiagnosis of radiculopathy. In (ed) Johnson, E. W., *Practical Electromyography* Second Edition. With permission.

the subsequent treatment program. Only when treatment decision making is impacted or when objective physiologic documentation is necessary should electrodiagnostic studies be considered.

3.4.3   Limitations of EMG

Although electrodiagnostic studies can be very helpful in the diagnosis of neuromuscular conditions, the needle EMG exam does possess some limitations. Needle electromyography only assesses motor nerves and so a pure sensory radiculopathy would not be detected. An EMG does not yield the specific cause for a condition. For instance, although the presence of an L5 radiculopathy can be determined in a worker, the cause of this L5 radiculopathy cannot be determined electrophysiologically. Whether it is from stenosis, a disc herniation, ischemia, or other etiologies, the cause cannot be determined based on the EMG/nerve conduction studies alone. Therefore, the electrodiagnostic studies must be combined with the history and physical and imaging studies. Also, the needle EMG will not identify where the root is compromised. The needle EMG will reveal the affected nerve root but will not precisely define where along the nerve root the problem is. Furthermore, electrodiagnostic study findings do not necessarily correlate with the subjective complaints of a patient. A mild electrophysiologic abnormality may be present in an individual with disabling low back and lower limb pain.

A negative needle EMG study does not imply that a patient is malingering. The electrodiagnostic study is a measure of neurophysiologic function. There are many other sources for limb symptoms which need to be ruled out. Limb pain may be referred from the joints, discs, muscles, or other tissues. Autonomic dysfunction is another source of limb symptoms that is not evaluated with standard EMG/nerve conduction studies. Furthermore, a false-negative needle EMG study may be obtained if too few muscles are sampled, which is an operator-dependent problem. A false-negative electrodiagnostic study may also be seen in a chronic radiculopathy where positive waves and fibrillation potentials have resolved. Usually, however, with careful motor unit action potential analysis the chronic radiculopathy will be recognized.

3.5   Electrodiagnostic Report

The electrodiagnostic report should include a brief introductory history and physical examination. It should include the neurophysiologic data, including nerve conduction study information with respect to distal latencies, action potential amplitude and duration, and nerve conduction velocities. The needle information should include data pertaining to insertional activity, the presence of positive waves and fibrillation potentials, and fasciculations, as well as information pertaining to the motor unit action potential analysis. This includes recruitment, amplitude, duration, and configuration of the motor unit action potentials. The information then needs to be interpreted by the electromyographer and a concise impression in simple neuromuscular terms should be included. The location and severity of the condition should be noted, as well as the chronicity and prognosis if possible. Ideally, if one limb is abnormal, the contralateral limb should be investigated and the results reported.

The electrodiagnostic report should be discussed with the referring physician. Recommendations for additional testing should be discussed with the referring physician. Some referring physicians appreciate recommendations included in the report, while others prefer this not be included. Below is a sample of a typical electrodiagnostic report:

PATIENT: Jim T.

DATE: 4-1-99

REFERRING PHYSICIAN: Dan K., M.D.

HISTORY: This is a 38-year-old male with a five-week history of low back pain and right lower limb pain radiating to the foot. There is associated tingling and weakness.

PHYSICAL EXAMINATION: Positive straight-leg raising. Negative crossed straight-leg raising. Manual muscle testing shows great toe extension at 4+/5, ankle dorsiflexion at 4+/5, and plantar flexion 5/5. Hypesthesias noted for the right lateral leg; otherwise normal. Examination for the left lower limb normal neurologically.

COMMENTS: The right sural nerve study shows a normal distal latency and sensory nerve action potential and duration. The right peroneal motor study shows a normal distal latency with a mild reduction in compound motor action potential amplitude compared to the normal left peroneal motor study. Peroneal motor nerve conduction velocity in the leg and across the knee is normal. Bilateral tibial H reflexes are within the normal limits.

The needle EMG shows 2 + positive waves and 1 + fibrillation potentials for the right gluteus medius, peroneus longus, extensor hallucis longus, and tibialis anterior muscles. There are 2 + positive waves and fibrillation potentials for the L5 paraspinal musculature on the right. With motor unit action potential analysis, recruitment is decreased to a mild degree in the L5 distribution with amplitude, duration, and configuration normal. The left-sided paraspinals and left lower limb muscles sampled were normal.

IMPRESSION: Acute right-sided L5 radiculopathy.

RECOMMENDATIONS: The patient is referred back to the referring physician for further evaluation and treatment.

3.6   Summary

The electrodiagnostic study is a valuable tool in the evaluation of individuals with neuromuscular disorders. It is particularly helpful when diagnosing workers with low back and lower limb pain. It is a sensitive dynamic test of physiologic function and therefore offers advantages over imaging studies which analyze anatomy only and have a high rate of false positive and false negative results. An EMG/NCS can localize, qualitate, and quantitate neurogenic disorders. It can determine the chronicity of neuronal injury and can assist the physician in prognostication. Electrodiagnostic abnormalities follow a temporal pattern and so EMG/NCS should be ordered with this information in mind.

3.7 References

1. Ball, R. Electrodiagnostic evaluation of the peripheral nervous system, in Delisa, J., ed., *Rehabilitation Medicine: Principles and Practice*. Philadelphia: Lippincott, 1988, 196–227.
2. Brown, W., Bolton, C., eds., *Clinical Electromyography*. Stoneham, MA: Butterworth Publishers, 1987.
3. Brown, W. F. *The Physiologic and Technical Basis of Electromyography*. Butterworth Publishers, 1984.
4. Chaudhry, V., Cornblath, D. R. Wallerian degeneration in human nerves. Presented at AAEM 38th Annual Scientific Meeting, Vancouver, British Columbia, September 28, 1991.
5. Chu-Andrews J., Johnson, R. J. *Electrodiagnosis: an anatomical and clinical approach*. Philadelphia: Lippincott, 1986.
6. Dawson, G. D., Merton, P. A. "Recurrent" discharges from motoneurons. XXth International Physiological Congress, Brussels, 1956.
7. Eccles, J. C. The central action of antidromic impulses in motor nerve fibers. *Pflugers Arch*. 260:385–415, 1955.
8. Fisher, M. A. AAEE Minimograph No. 13: Physiology and clinical use of the F response. AAEE, 1980.
9. Frank, L. W., Schneider, D. S., Zuhosky, J. P. Anatomic and technical considerations in needle electromyography of the lumbar spine, in Kraft, G. H., Wertsch, J. J., eds., *Physical Medicine and Rehabilitation Clinics in North America*, 9:795–814, 1998.
10. Haig, A. J., Talley, C., Grobler, L. J. et al. Paraspinal mapping: Quantified needle electromyography in lumbar radiculopathy. *Muscle Nerve* 16:477–484, 1993.
11. Hitselberger, W., Witten, R. Abnormal myelograms in asymptomatic patients. *Neurosurgery* 28:204–206, 1968.
12. Johnson, E. W., ed., *Practical Electromyography*, Second Edition. Baltimore: Williams & Wilkins, 1988, 231–233.
13. Khatri, B., Baruah, J., McQuillen, M. Correlation of electromyography with computed tomography in evaluation of lower back pain. *Arch. Neurol*. 4:594–597, 1984.
14. Kimura, J. *Electrodiagnosis in Diseases of Nerve and Muscle: Principles and Practice*, Second Edition. Philadelphia: F. A. Davis, 1989.
15. Kraft, G. H. Fibrillation potential amplitude and muscle atrophy following peripheral nerve injury. *Muscle & Nerve* 1990:13:814–821.
16. Lajoie, W. Nerve root compression: Correlation of electromyographic, myelographic, and surgical findings. *Arch. Phys. Med. Rehab*. 53:390–392, 1972.

17. Lauder, T. D., Dillingham, T. R., Huston, C. W. et al. Lumbosacral radiculopa-
     thy screen: Optimizing the number of muscles studied. *Am. J. Phys. Med.
     Rehabil.* 73:394–402, 1994.
18. Loyd, D. P. C. The interaction of antidromic and orthodromic volleys in a seg-
     mental spinal motor nucleus. *Neurophysiol.* 6:143–151, 1943.
19. Magladery J., McDougal, D. B. Electrophysiological studies of nerve and reflex
     activity in normal man. Identification of certain reflexes in the electromyogram
     and the conduction velocity of peripheral nerve fibers. *Bull. Johns Hopkins Hosp.*
     86:265–290, 1950.
20. Mayer, R. F., Feldman, R. G. Observations on the nature of the F-wave in man.
     Neurology 17:147–156, 1967.
21. McLeod, J. G., Wray, S. H. An experimental study of the F-wave in the baboon.
     Neurol. Neurosurg. Psychiatry 29:196–200, 1966.
22. Miller, R. G. AAEE Minimonograph No. 28: Injury to peripheral nerves. *Muscle
     & Nerve* 10:698–710, 1987.
23. Pope, M., Anderson, G., Frymoyer, J. et al. *Occupational Low Back Pain,
     Assessment, Treatment, and Prevention.* St. Louis: Mosby, 1991.
24. Renshaw, B. Influence of discharge of motoneurons upon excitation of neigh-
     boring motoneurons. *Neurophysiol.* 4:167–183, 1941.
25. Seddon, H. J. Three types of nerve injury. *Brain* 1943; 66:236–288.
26. Stalberg, E. V, Trontelj, J. V. *Single Fiber Electromyography:* Old Working Mirvalle
     Press, 1979, 1–224.
27. Wertsch, J. J., Mauldin, C. C., Melvin, J. L. et al. A focal late response in a central
     cervical disc. *Muscle & Nerve* 12:758, 1989.
28. Wilbourn, A., Aminoff, M. The electrophysiologic examination in patients with
     radiculopathies. *Muscle & Nerve* 1:1099–1114, 1988.

chapter four

Diagnostic Spinal Injections for Low Back Pain

Jeffrey L. Woodward, M.D.,
Robert E. Windsor, M.D.

4.1   Overview

The use of diagnostic spinal injections has become an integral part of low back pain management for the diagnosis of specific active pain generators in these pain patients. A specific diagnosis of the origin of a patient's spine pain contributes to the treating physician's ability to determine the most reasonable course of treatment for that patient's prognosis. The increasing reliance on fluoroscopy during diagnostic spine injections has allowed for much more precise needle placement during the injections and more accurate diagnosis.

4.2   Diagnostic Evaluations

Several factors play an important role in the clinical utility of diagnostic spinal injections. First, pain in the low back and lower extremities can have very similar, if not identical, location and quality despite anatomically different pain generators in different patients. In addition, provocative maneuvers on physical examination have yet to reveal any accurate diagnostic information in the identification of specific spine pain generators. Imaging studies, such as CT and MRI scans, are known to reveal obvious structural abnormalities in the lumbar spine in asymptomatic volunteers indicating that the presence of such abnormalities in no way confirms that a symptomatic patient's symptoms originate from that structural abnormality.[7, 92]

One important consideration in the interpretation of diagnostic spine injections is the well-documented occurrence of placebo response which seems to be especially prominent in the initial spine injection. A placebo response is more likely to be seen in patients who are positive responders at least briefly to most treatments offered by the physician including oral medications and physical therapy, but does not necessarily correlate to long-term response or benefit. A brief placebo response to a diagnostic anesthetic spine injection can lead to an incorrect diagnosis regarding the origin of the patient's active spine pain. For example, the placebo response to a single anesthetic facet joint injection has been recently reported at 32–38%.[77] One procedural technique that has been proposed to delineate physiologic pain relief from a placebo response is the use of successive spine injections using local anesthetics with significantly different duration of action. Typically, the double block paradigm involves performing the initial spine injection with lidocaine, and if a positive response is reported, then the same procedure is performed at a later date using bupivacaine. Based on the duration of action of these two anesthetics, physiologic pain relief following anesthetic injection would typically last significantly longer following bupivacaine as compared to lidocaine.[29] However, there are limitations to dual medial branch blocks because some patients respond on placebo challenge even when there is time contingent relief. The comparative blocks cannot replace a placebo injection but do decrease the false positive rate.[61] Also, placebo responses are known to attenuate with repeated applications of the same treatment, and in this way, serial anesthetic injection at the same anatomic site which is providing physiologic pain relief should demonstrate no such attenuation in effect.

Since this textbook is focusing on the treatment of work-related injuries, some consideration as to the validity of pain responses reported by patients involved in the Workers' Compensation system often associated with some monetary secondary gain should be considered. One study revealed that the short-term pain response of patients having apparent low back pain and sympathetically mediated pain in the lower extremity was not related in any way to their Workers' Compensation status. In that study, generalized poor response to the injection, and other treatments, were correlated specifically only with the level of the patient's pain behaviors such as learned helplessness, low degrees of personal sense of responsibility, and an exaggerated amount of pain focused behavior.[15]

In work-related low back pain patients, unwavering complaints of significant low back and/or leg pain which is not responsive at all to aggressive nonsurgical treatments is often encountered. The physician's assessment of the patient's response to a spine injection is often very helpful in providing insight into the patient's pain tolerance and pain and stress management capabilities. The spinal injection provides the physician with an opportunity to observe the patient during procedures with familiar pain stimuli such as local anesthetic injection, and an experienced physician can gauge an individual patient's pain response to that familiar pain stimulus as compared to the average or routine response to that stimulus. Assessment of the patient's overall level of anxiety during the procedure can also give the practitioner some sense of the patient's underlying psychological status. Connally and Sanders studied sympathetic nerve injections and found a definite correlation between the presence of abnormal overt pain behavior exhibited by patients at the first injection with a poor overall outcome of both the injections themselves and general response to an interdisciplinary pain management treatment program.[20] The overt exaggerated pain behaviors observed during spinal injection were more closely correlated to a poor clinical recovery than was testing of the patient's cognitive pain coping abilities, number of previous back surgeries, or the presence of secondary economic compensation for that back condition.

The following sections will present information regarding diagnostic spinal injections only, while the therapeutic aspects of these injections will be discussed in the next chapter. Diagnostic information from spinal injections can be obtained from both the patient's immediate response to local anesthetic, as well as the delayed response to locally injected corticosteroids. More controlled and precise diagnostic information is obtained by the immediate response to local anesthetics. However, the patient must be experiencing a significant amount of low back or leg pain immediately preceding the anesthetic injection in order to obtain diagnostic information from the injection. For example, patients with milder radicular symptoms may have intermittent leg pain and a diagnostic anesthetic selective nerve root block would have to be postponed if the patient was not having the typical leg pain at the time of the scheduled injection. For diagnostic information obtained from the more delayed response to corticosteroids, however, the patient does not necessarily have to be experiencing the typical back or leg discomfort right at the time of steroid infiltration. The diagnostic information would be gained from the patient's pain response within the one- to two-week period following the steroid injection.

As mentioned above, the use of fluoroscopy during diagnostic spinal injections is necessary to achieve the specific localization of needle placement required for selective infiltration of both local anesthetics and corticosteroid solutions. For lumbar facet joint and sacroiliac injections, the joint spaces are narrow and often irregular, with a great deal of individual variability in joint orientation making fluoroscopy essential in achieving reliable intraarticular needle placement.

For transforaminal epidural steroid injections, accurate localization of the needle within the lumbar neuroforamen also necessitates the use of fluoroscopy which will provide documentation as to the proximity of the injectate to the nerve root sleeve as well as the amount of injectate flow through the foramen into the central spinal canal. Obviously, use of fluroscopy also eliminates the possibility of an inadvertent intravascular injection of local anesthetic greatly reducing the risks for these procedures. Lumbar sympathetic blockade has been performed routinely by anesthesiologists without fluoroscopy for many years, however, the use of fluoroscopy allows the injectionist to document the specific location of needle placement and distribution of injectate. In patients who have no significant pain relief or change in temperature of the affected limb from lumbar sympathetic anesthetic injection, fluoroscopy would allow the physician to more confidently interpret the negative response as being due to the absence of a sympathetic origin of the patient's pain instead of due to inaccurate localization of the anesthetic, thereby improving the diagnostic potential of this procedure.

Interpretation of the patient's response to local anesthetic injection with diagnostic spinal blocks is an essential part of these procedures. The use of pre- and postinjection pain diagrams and visual analog scale pain assessment is often helpful in documenting the patient's response. There is no clearly accepted guideline as to the level of pain relief which is required after anesthetic injection to consider the injection as having provided a diagnostic positive response. Ideally, 100% pain relief is obtained and the results of the block are easily interpreted. However, many spine injections result in only partial pain relief of a patient's typical back or leg pain. In addition, acute pain from the injection itself can confound the diagnostic result of the block, especially in the evaluation of focal pain such as facet and SI joint injections. Some studies propose that 75% pain relief is adequate to consider the spine structure anesthetized as a significant pain generator with a more recent facet joint article recommending a 90% pain relief threshold. Performing pre- and postprocedure physical examination of the patient is also helpful including repeating any provocative or stress maneuvers to the spine which reliably aggravated the patient's pain prior to injection. As discussed previously, placebo response and/or false positive response to a single anesthetic injection in the spine must always be considered.

4.3   Facet Joint Injections

Lumbar facet joints have been proposed for many years as a possible source of acute and chronic pain in the lumbar spine.[25] The actual prevalence of facet or zygapophyseal (Z) joint pain has been quite variable and cited in one recent review to range from 7.7 to 75%, although many of the previous studies have been poorly controlled.[26] It is clear from diagnostic injection studies, however, that the lumbar Z-joint can be a source of both acute and chronic low back pain.[9, 75] Controlled studies using comparative blocks and placebo control blocks have yielded a prevalence of this condition at 15 to 40%.[76, 78]

The best diagnostic test available to identify active lumbar Z-joint pain is pain relief from anesthetic injection into the Z-joint or to the nerve innervating these joints. There is no portion of the patient's history or physical examination testing which reliably identifies patients having Z-joint pain.[76, 78] Imaging studies which reveal structural abnormalities of the lumbar Z-joints also have no diagnostic value in identifying patients with active Z-joint pain. Weisel et al. found that over 50% of asymptomatic individuals greater than 40 years of age had evidence of lumbar facet joint arthropathy on lumbar spine CT scan.[92] In a more recent study, patients having CT scan Z-joint abnormalities underwent Z-joint anesthetic injection under fluoroscopic guidance and no significant correlation was noted between the scan results and the diagnostic injection results.[79] In the most recent review by Bogduk, he reiterates that Z-joint pain cannot be identified reliably by the history, physical exam, plain radiography, CT or SPECT scan, and that anesthetic injection under fluoroscopy is necessary to make the accurate diagnosis of Z-joint pain.[4, 61] Part of the difficulty in identifying Z-joint pain from history and physical exam is the variable pain distribution originating from the Z-joint. Pain referral patterns associated with Z-joint pain have been shown to most commonly involve localized pain in the vicinity of the painful joint. However, referred pain and even paresthesias into the ipsilateral lower extremity has been documented, as well as nondermatomal extremity sensory alteration and even pain-inhibited weakness.[66, 76] Pain provocation with reproducible referral patterns has also been reported in studies of asymptomatic individuals injected with solution into the lumbar Z-joints with associated joint capsule distention.[66]

A recent well-controlled study evaluating patients with a diagnosis of chronic low back pain receiving both lumbar Z-joint injection and discography to carefully diagnose the source of lumbar spine pain reported that 15% of these patients had significant Z-joint pain. This was using dual comparative facet and/or medial branch blocks.[76] A later study utilizing placebo controlled blocks and their response to fluoroscopically guided Z-joint anesthetic injection reported 40% of patients with a diagnosis of lumbar Z-joint pain.[78] The actual prevalence of Z-joint pain would no doubt vary somewhat based on the specific patient population that was being studied and may vary between different physicians clinical patient population.

Previous studies indicate that the most accurate method of diagnosing lumbar Z-joint pain is with differential anesthetic injections using fluoroscopy comparing the patient's duration of pain response to lidocaine with that from longer acting bupivacaine (Figure 4.1).[9, 76] It has also been demonstrated that no correlation exists between pain provocation during Z-joint intra-articular injection and low back pain originating from those Z-joints which is relieved with Z-joint anesthetic injection.[56] Bogduk in a recent presentation of Z-joint injection procedural techniques indicates that lumbar Z-joint pain diagnosis can be adequately achieved either with local anesthetic infiltration in the Z-joint or anesthetic nerve block of the medial branches of the dorsal rami that innervate the target facet joint.[9] Bogduk also suggests that not all of the patient's low back discomfort need be relieved by Z-joint injection to diagnose Z-joint pain since there may also be co-existing pain generators. However, he does indicate that the patient should have at least 90% pain relief in a distinct region of pain corresponding to the anatomic location of that particular Z-joint. A very significant false positive diagnostic block rate of 32 to 38% has been identified to occur with initial single Z-joint anesthetic injection.[77] Again, the false positive response can be more accurately identified with use of serial anesthetic blocks. A false negative rate of

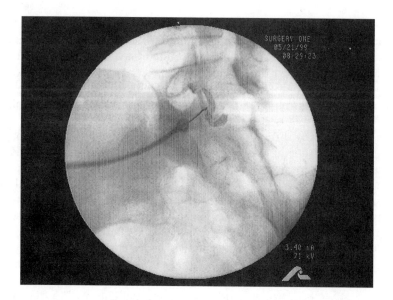

Figure 4.1   Lumbar Z-joint injection with contrast and fluoroscopy. With permission.

about 8% has been identified with medial branch nerve injection which appears to be due to the uptake of local anesthetic occurring with inadvertent intravenous injection which can occur even with correct anatomic needle placement and can be avoided by the use of contrast under fluoroscopy.[9, 30, 56] Identification of false positive responses to Z-joint injections is important prior to recommending the more invasive neuroablative procedures involving the medial branch of the dorsal ramus denervation techniques.

Previous diagnostic spine injection studies have reported that it is unusual for an individual patient to have significant active pain from both the Z-joints and also from either the sacroiliac joint or lumbar disc at the same time.[77] Also, it has been reported that typically Z-joint pain will occur from only one segmental level at any given time, however, pain originating from bilateral Z-joints at the same level is not unusual.[78]

Lumbar facet or Z-joints are the posterolateral articulations between the vertebral bodies. Each Z-joint is a true synovial joint. The fibrous Z-joint capsule has extensions just beyond the superior and inferior bony margins of the joint forming two subcapsular recesses.[66] These subcapsular recesses can often be accessed with a needle to allow intra-articular infiltration if the main portion of the joint is inaccessible. Each lumbar Z-joint is innervated by medial branches of the primary dorsal rami (MBDR) which exit from the neural foramen at that segmental level and from the foramen at the level above that Z-joint. The L1-L4 MBDR branches travel laterally out of the neural foramen and over the superior border of the most medial portion of the transverse process and proceed inferiorly and medially eventually crossing over the adjacent lamina. Typically, the MBDR nerve runs under the mamillary ligament located at the junction of the transverse process with the superior articulating process.[8] For the L5-S1 Z-joint, the target nerve is not the medial branch but the actual L5 dorsal ramus which travels between the superior articulating process of L5 and the sacral ala below. Additional innervation to the L5-S1 facet joint may enter the joint from the inferior aspect with nerves that exit the spinal canal from the ipsilateral S1 foramen.[24]

Lumbar Z-joint injections are done with the patient in the prone position. The procedure must be done with contrast and fluoroscopy unless contraindicated. Diagnostic Z-joint injections may be done using only local anesthetic solution. A total volume of 0.5 to 1.0 ml anesthetic and/or steroid is injected with the volume limited to avoid joint capsular rupture. Due to the small volume of anesthetic injected, more definitive analgesic responses are often obtained by using a higher concentration of local anesthetic such as lidocaine 2% or 4% or bupivacaine 0.5%.

MBDR anesthetic injections are also performed under fluoroscopy. To anesthetize a specific Z-joint, the MBDR blocks must be done at the two levels adjacent to that Z-joint (Figures 4.2 and 4.3). For example, to anesthetize

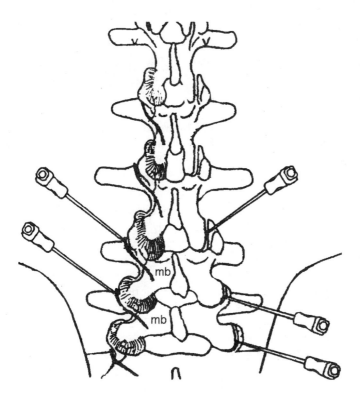

Figure 4.2 Injections for the medial branch of the primary dorsal ramus (medial branch block). From Bogduk, N.: Back Pain: Zygapophyseal Blocks and Epidural Steroids, in *Neural Blockade in Clinical Anesthesia and Management of Pain*, Second Edition, Cousins M. J., Bridenbaugh P.O., eds. New York: Lippincott Co., 1988. With permission.

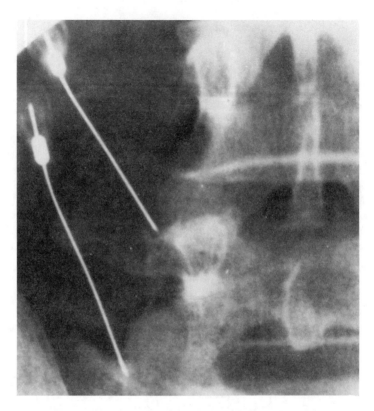

Figure 4.3   The L4 medial branch and L5 dorsal ramus are blocked under fluo-roscopy, From Dreyfuss, P., Lagattuta, F., Kaplansky, B. and Heller, B., *Zygapophyseal Joint Injection Techniques in the Spinal Axis*. In Lennard, T. ed. *Physiatric Procedures in Clinical Practice*. Philadelphia: Hanley and Belfus Inc., 1995 with permission.

the L4-5 Z-joint, the L3 MBDR must be blocked at the L4 transverse process and the L4 MBDR at the transverse process of L5. Because the L5-S1 Z-joint may receive additional innervation inferiorly from nerves exiting the S1 fora-men, these branches can be blocked just above the S1 posterior foramina.[24] Initial venous uptake is associated with a 50% false-negative response, de-spite repositioning and subsequent lack of venous uptake. If venous uptake is avoided, Kaplan has demonstrated an 89% sensitivity using only two me-dial branch nerve injections for each targeted joint.[56]

Typically, no specific premedication, IV access or vital sign monitoring is required for either Z-joint intra-articular or MBDR anesthetic injection. Side effects are usually limited to brief discomfort at the injection site, although more serious vasovagal and allergic reactions are possible and resuscitative equipment and support should be readily available. The patient is examined after the procedure to document the pain response and then is ready for dis-charge if no complications are identified.

4.4 Sacroiliac Joint Injections

The prevalence and importance of the sacroiliac joint (SI joint) as a pain generator and source of low back pain and impairment has been reviewed extensively of late without definitive conclusions.[27, 74] Many previous studies on SI joint pain have had little in the way of experimental controls. Recently, more reliable access to the SI joint for diagnostic anesthetic injection has been standardized and used as an indicator of active SI joint pain. As with lumbar facet joint pain, no physical exam technique or provocative maneuver has been shown to reliably diagnose patients having SI joint pain.[27, 63, 74, 84] Pain originating from the SI joint has been reported as having the potential to cause pain not only in the posterior ipsilateral sacral region, but also in a variety of referred pain patterns including into the buttocks, groin, thigh, and even calf and foot discomfort.[74] It is also assumed that, similar to other adjacent spinal structures, structural abnormalities in the SI joint seen on plain X-ray or CT scanning may or may not be correlated with active pain from that SI joint.[27]

Despite previous reports of referred pain from SI joint pathology, most studies indicate that an active SI joint problem is accompanied by significant pain localized to the SI joint region.[36] Patients that have maximal pain below L5 and have pain and the sacral sulcus or point to the posterior superior iliac spine as their pain source, do have intra-articular pain as judged by SI joint injections with a positive predictive value of approximately 60%.[29, 84] Consideration of the SI joint as a significant contributor to any patient's low back pain should be given if the patient's maximum pain is located just inferior to the posterior-superior iliac spine and over the SI joint area. One recent study indicated that patients with unilateral SI joint pain that was confirmed by fluoroscopic guided SI joint anesthetic injection typically reported their region of maximum pain in a 3 cm wide by 10 cm long region beginning just below the PSIS.[35] One other experimental technique to study SI joint pain referral patterns is the injection of fluid into the joint to distend the joint and capsule. Fortin performed SI injection on 10 asymptomatic volunteers and describes complaints of unsustained "pressure" discomfort from these individuals during the injection into the asymptomatic SI joint.[36] A marked distinction is made with regard to the pain response noted with symptomatic SI joint injections which was described as sustained intense gluteal pain. In addition, patients with only unilateral SI joint pain who underwent bilateral SI joint injections described this intense pain in the affected joint but only transient milder discomfort or pressure with injection in the asymptomatic SI joint. The most common pain pattern from SI joint infiltration involved pain localized to the ipsilateral SI joint region and the most common referred pain radiated to the ipsilateral groin.[34] Dreyfuss has reported that the presence of provocative pain with SI joint infiltration has no correlation with subsequent pain relief.[29] Derby has reported a number of patients with concordant pain on SI joint injection followed by unconvincing pain relief from anesthetic injection resulting in an uncertain diagnosis of SI joint pain.[22]

The actual prevalence of SI joint pain is uncertain at this time. Aprill studied patients with chronic low back pain and found that 15% had pain originating solely from the SI joint based on significant pain relief from SI joint anesthetic injection.[3] Another study performing SI joint injection on patients having pain localized to the sacrum below the L5-S1 level noted a positive response to SI joint anesthetic injection in 30% (13/43) of the patients studied.[74] Schwarzer found that in patients having maximum pain specifically localized to the SI joint region, a total of 30% (16/54) of these patients had significant pain relief with anesthetic SI joint injection indicating that the majority of patients with pain well-localized to the SI joint do not have pain originating from that joint. The patient's immediate pain relief from anesthetic SI joint injection as noted is an important diagnostic consideration however, the delayed response to corticosteroids should also be considered especially in patients suspected of having a significant inflammatory component to the possible SI joint pain.

SI joint injections under fluoroscopy can also be helpful in diagnosing structural abnormalities to the joint. Following SI joint arthrograms with contrast, contralateral oblique, PA and lateral X-ray views can identify a variety of SI joint deformities such as joint capsule diverticula and frank joint capsular tears. No prior SI joint study has shown a correlation between provocation of pain with SI joint injection and structural abnormalities seen on postarthrogram imaging tests. CT scanning of the postarthrogram SI joint can also be performed within one to two hours after injection which will identify anterior SI joint capsular defects especially well.[37] The lumbosacral trunk is immediately anterior to the anterior sacroiliac joint capsule. The ventral sacroiliac ligament anterior capsular complex has been demonstrated on magnetic resonance images to be only 2 mm in thickness.[55] Of note, three possible physical communication pathways between the SI intra-articular space and adjacent neural pathways have been identified with a proposal that leakage of inflammatory mediators from the SI joint after injury with direct communication to the S1 nerve root may explain the anecdotal cases of radicular pain secondary to SI joint injury.[37]

The SI joint is considered a synovial joint which varies greatly with respect to size, shape, and contour between individuals. Only a portion of the joint has a true synovial structure which is most consistently located at the S2 vertebral level, but may extend from S1 to S3 and typically lies in the anterior-inferior 1/2 to 2/3 segment of the joint.[85] The inferior aspect of the SI joint has become the most accepted portion of the joint for needle penetration and arthrography. The posterior border of the SI joint is formed by the relatively thick posterior sacroiliac ligaments. The posterior ligament is often incomplete with intermittent rents or openings, but has been identified as a very strong ligamentous structure. The anterior SI joint ligament is usually

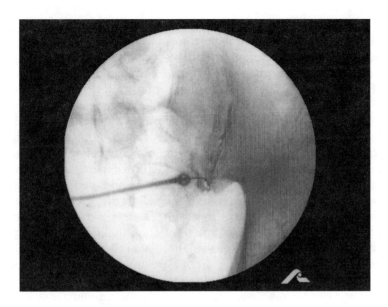

Figure 4.4 Sacroiliac joint arthrogram. With permission.

continuous with the anterior joint capsule and is considered to be relatively weak.[6] The diffuse regional innervation of the SI joint has been recently reviewed thoroughly and has been implicated to explain the variety of pain referral patterns thought to be associated with SI joint pathology.[26, 27, 37]

Due to the great individual variability in the structure and alignment of the SI joint, reliable intra-articular needle placement requires fluoroscopic imaging. The recommended target entry site into the joint is 1 to 2 cm above the inferior osseous border of the posterior SI joint.[27] Dreyfuss recommends the use of a .22-guage spinal needle to negotiate the posterior SI joint ligament. An arthrogram appearance confirms needle placement with injection of 0.3 to 0.5 cc of non-ionic contrast (Figure 4.4). Following contrast, either lidocaine or bupivacaine can be injected to anesthetize the joint prior to postinjection evaluation.

4.5 Lumbar Transforaminal Epidural Injections

Therapeutic epidural steroid injection has been an accepted part of spine pain treatment for many years.[95] Selective lumbar epidural procedures done for diagnostic purposes has evolved more recently associated with the increasing reliance on fluoroscopy and improving precision with these injections.

Transforaminal or selective nerve root injections can be used to provide diagnostic information in patients presented with a lumbosacral radiculopathy.[83] Pain relief from radicular symptoms following transforaminal injection can be used to diagnose whether or not a specific nerve root is causing pain as well as help predict surgical outcomes. The need for such diagnostic procedures for epidural pathology is necessary due to the poor correlation between structural abnormalities identified on imaging studies such as CT and MRI scanning and the actual pain generator of low back and radicular pain.[7, 92] Also, radicular pain patterns for a specific nerve root can vary significantly between individual patients. The most common scenarios requiring diagnostic nerve root injections are in postsurgical patients with more than one segmental level revealing postsurgical or structural abnormalities, as well as older patients with significant structural degenerative changes visualized at multiple levels.[47, 50] In particular, the anesthetic selective nerve root injection can be helpful in distinguishing L3 from L4 nerve root pain and most commonly L5 from S1 nerve root pain. The use of the diagnostic nerve root injection can help correlate structural abnormalities seen on imaging studies with the patient's pain presentation, as well as isolate the symptomatic nerve root prior to pursuing surgical treatments. Therapeutic spine injection including midline and translaminar posterior epidural steroid injections and caudal injections have no selective or segmental diagnostic information due to the likely spread of injectate from these approaches to two or three spinal levels.

For diagnostic selective nerve root anesthetic injections, the patient's preinjection distribution and quality of pain can be recorded by pain diagram and physical examination. Following the injection, the patient is then reexamined including provocative testing such as straight leg raising for comparison to preprocedure results. As with the other anesthetic spine injections, significant short-term relief of radicular extremity pain would indicate that the target nerve root was the active pain generator. Incomplete relief of radicular pain following anesthetic injection makes a definitive diagnosis more difficult; however, relief of 75–90% of radicular pain following nerve root anesthetic injection is strongly suggestive of at least a significant portion of the patient's pain originating from the nerve root at that level. Haueisen also suggested that exact recreation of the patient's typical radicular pain with needle placement adjacent to the nerve root also provides an indication that the nerve is a significant pain generator.[47]

Herron reported a significant correlation between leg pain relief, even if temporary, secondary to steroid nerve root injection and an increased chance of good surgical outcome for patients with disc herniation, bony stenosis, or postsurgical radicular pain.[50] Haueisen performed selective anesthetic nerve root injections using fluoroscopy and 1 ml of 1% lidocaine and considered a positive response to be associated with complete postinjection leg pain relief, relief of straight leg raise abnormality, and no pain when standing or walking.[47] In his patient group with total pain relief following a single level nerve root injection, 93% of these patients had clearly visible nerve root injury at that level at the time of direct visualization of the nerve during subsequent surgery. Of the 55 patients with positive selective nerve root injections, 29% were pain-free following subsequent surgery, 20% had only slight residual pain, 32% had mild pain, and the remaining 18% had moderate to severe residual pain. More recently, Derby et al. showed the significant negative predictive value of transforaminal corticosteroid injections in relation to the surgical outcome for the treatment of chronic radiculopathy.[23] Of the 38 patients with radicular pain for at least 12 months receiving less than 80% leg pain relief one week after selective nerve root block with corticosteroid, only 2 of the 38 had significant relief following surgery for their radicular pain. In the same study, 11 of 13 patients with significant pain relief following steroid nerve root block noted a positive surgical outcome.[23] Another study evaluated patients having unilateral radicular pain from bony neural foraminal stenosis. Of the 19 patients who had complete leg pain relief following lidocaine nerve root block and undergoing subsequent decompressive foraminotomy, 16 reported a good surgical response with "considerable" pain relief.[87]

Diagnostic transforaminal anesthetic and steroid injections can have an effect on the posterior annular fibers of the intervertebral disc via the sinuvertebral nerve, as well as an effect on the exiting nerve root at the level of the injection. The intervertebral neuroforamina is bordered superiorly and inferiorly by the pedicles of the adjacent vertebra, anteriorly by the posterior border of the disc, and posteriorly by the adjacent zygapophyseal joint capsule. In the lumbar spine, the nerve roots travel inferiorly and exit in essentially a lateral plane without significant anterior or posterior angulation near the foramen and exit just under the superior pedicle with a downward course of 40–50 from horizontal. The nerve root and associated vascular structures typically occupy the superior portion of each foramen. Just proximal to the exiting nerve root within the neuroforamen is the dorsal root ganglion which is at some risk of needle contact during transforaminal injections. A sleeve of dura surrounds each nerve root as it exits through the neuroforamen with a gradual thinning of the dural sleeve distally. Just distal to the dorsal root ganglion are the dorsal and ventral nerve roots which then merge to form the spinal nerve to which the dura matter adheres directly becoming continuous with the epineurium. Within the neuroforamen, segmental radicular arteries enter the spine and pass through the dura within the foramen at the region of the thinned dural cuff and connect to the anterior spinal artery. Most of these radicular arteries are quite small and supply only a minimal portion of the total spinal cord arterial blood flow at that level. Associated venous structures also travel adjacent to the nerve root in the foramen making direct intravascular injection with a transforaminal needle approach possible.

Accurate localization of the needle tip into the lumbar neuroforamina adjacent to an exiting nerve root requires fluoroscopic guidance (Figures 4.5 and 4.6). The dye pattern may reveal pathology in the area of the exiting nerve root such as abnormal position and course of the nerve secondary to compressive vertebral osteophytes or a lateral disc herniation.[23]

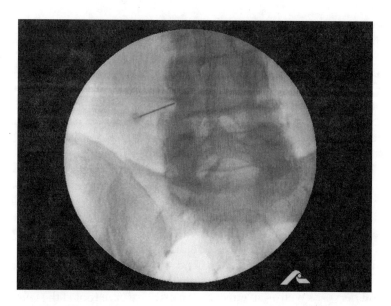

Figure 4.5   Needle placement for left L4 transforaminal injection. With permission.

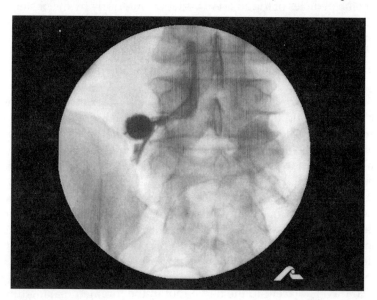

Figure 4.6   Lumbar transforaminal (selective nerve root block) injection with fluoroscopy. With permission.

The most serious complication from transforaminal selective nerve root injection aside from the general complications of vasovagal and allergic reactions is direct needle contact with the exiting nerve root. The transforaminal approach must be done very carefully with a slow advancement of the needle and verbal communication with the patient during the injection to identify quickly the development of radicular paresthesias or pain as the needle approaches the nerve root. The hand holding the needle should be braced against the patient's back so that the needle will not be advanced more deeply if the patient unexpectedly moves or rises from the table. The use of fluoroscopy should eliminate any risk of direct intravascular injection with careful monitoring of fluoroscopic images during contrast injection. The volume of local anesthetics injected with the transforaminal approach as described above does not approach published toxic levels for these anesthetics typically necessary to cause CNS or cardiac toxicity, but vasovagal and allergic reactions are possible.

No widely accepted patient monitoring guidelines are established specifically for transforaminal anesthetic steroid injections. Preprocedure IV access is advisable but not mandatory and local community standards should be followed. As with other injections, advanced cardiopulmonary resuscitative equipment and personnel should be readily available.

4.6 Lumbar Sympathetic Nerve Injections

Lumbar sympathetic nerve injection is probably the least common lumbosacral injection performed for diagnostic purposes. Sympathetic injections are classically recommended for treatment of suspected sympathetic mediated pain (SMP) associated with symptoms of burning pain, discomfort increased with light tactile stimulation, signs of altered sympathetic nervous tone including local erythema, edema, altered skin temperature, skin discoloration, and possible dystrophic changes to the skin and nails.[11] SMP conditions in the lower extremities can develop most commonly after traumatic injuries including those associated with lumbar radiculopathy. Lower extremity SMP has also been reported following lumbosacral spine surgery.[93]

In patients with SMP associated with lumbosacral radiculopathy, diagnostic, and therapeutic anesthetic, and/or corticosteroid injections at the specific nerve roots consistent with the patient's radicular pain may provide adequate diagnosis and relief of the patient's SMP. If not, then specific lumbar sympathetic blockade may be advisable. The sympathetic block can help answer the question of whether the patient specifically has pain mediated through the sympathetic nervous system, but it will not localize pathology to any specific lumbar level. A successful sympathetic injection results in changes to sympathetic nerve function without significantly altering somatic nerve function. For example, following a sympathetic block, there should be relief of sympathetic discomfort without concurrent changes in somatic sensation as indicated by a normal postinjection sensory exam and minimal effects on lower extremity pain threshold testing. Successful sympathetic blockage is most commonly documented by a postinjection increase in skin temperature of 2–3 Cs.[11] Windsor indicates that a positive response should include pain relief of 75% or more particularly of dysaesthetic pain in the absence of somatic blockade.[93] As with other spine injections, placebo responses are possible, but consistent significant pain relief to repeated sympathetic blocks would diminish the likelihood of confounding placebo response.

The sympathetic nerve trunks in the lumbar spine run longitudinally along the bilateral anterolateral surfaces of the vertebral bodies from L1 to L5 (Figure 4.7). The lumbar sympathetic chains are in direct connection to the thoracic and pelvic sympathetic nerves. In the lumbar spine, the sympathetic nerve ganglia are located just anterior to the prevertebral fascia of the psoas muscle. The exact number and location of sympathic chain ganglia in the lumbar spine varies considerably from one individual to another and can also vary from side to side in the same person.[11] Most commonly, the sympathetic ganglia are clumped between the L2 and L4 vertebral bodies with the ganglia ranging in size from 3–5 mm wide to 10–15 mm long. Most of the lumbar sympathic fibers traveling inferiorly from the lumbar spine into the lower extremities pass through the L2 and L3 region ganglia and injection of anesthetic at these levels can usually invoke complete sympathic denervation of the ipsilateral lower extremity.[89] Previously, anesthetic injection at two lumbar levels has been recommended for reliable complete lower extremity sympathetic blockade and typically performed at the L1 to L2 level, as well as at the L4 level.[11] Major vascular structures are located usually just anterior and medial to the lumbar sympathetic chains with the inferior vena cava traveling just right of midline and the aorta usually at or just left of midline anterior to the vertebral body. The exact relationship between these major vessels and the lumbar sympathetic chain can be quite variable.[11, 13]

Lumbar sympathetic injections should be performed with fluoroscopy for precise localization and to decrease the risk of an intravascular injection.

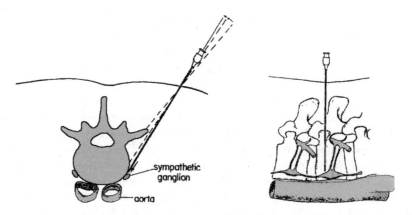

Figure 4.7a   Technique for lumbar sympathetic block at L2. With permission.

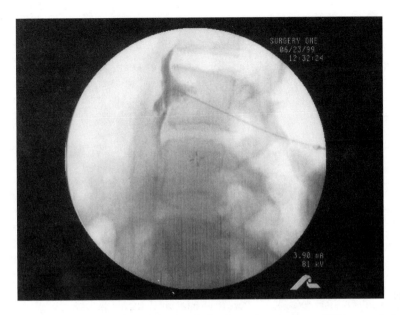

Figure 4.7b Lumbar sympathetic block with fluoroscopic guidance. With permission.

Following lumbar sympathetic anesthetic injection, the patient must be monitored closely for both clinical response and side effects. One study indicated that the maximum serum concentration of bupivacaine following lumbar sympathetic injection occurred 10 to 45 minutes following the injection with a mean of 24 minutes. They noted that after injection of 30 cc 0.175% bupivacaine, none of their patients developed any clinical signs of CNS toxicity or toxic serum levels of bupivacaine.[96] After the injection, the ipsilateral lower extremity is monitored for temperature and skin color changes to clinically identify a successful sympathetic block, as well as a reexamination to document lower extremity pain relief 30–45 minutes following the injection. With regard to patient monitoring, IV access is mandatory for lumbar sympathetic injections due to the much larger volume of anesthetic used as compared to the other diagnostic injections discussed in this section. Continuous blood pressure and pulse monitoring should be performed as well. Complications can arise such as significant hypotension which can develop from the sympathetic blockade during the injection, as well as systemic side effects from the close proximity of large vascular structures to the target injection site. The patient should be monitored for a minimum of 60 minutes following the injection before release from an outpatient setting. Other complications reported from lumbar sympathetic injections include lumbar nerve plexus injection, renal puncture, intralymphatic injection and genitofemoral neuralgia.[48, 93]

4.7   Lumbar Discography

In 1858, Luschka described the herniated intervertebral disc.[62] In 1934, Mixter and Barr described the connection between the herniated disc and radiculopathy.[65] Since 1934 there has been an intense focus on the lumbar disc as a source of back and lower extremity pain. The pathogenesis and natural history of lumbar disc injury have been described.[1, 5, 16, 21, 32, 33, 54, 57, 64, 70, 71, 72, 91]

In 1929, Schmorl was the first to perform a disc injection.[73] In 1938, Steindler used the injection of procaine into the disc to relieve low back pain and in 1948 Hirsch and Lindblom, in two separate studies, noted that the injection of a herniated disc caused an intense exacerbation of pain.[51, 60, 88] In 1951, Wise and Weiford were the first to inject a disc in the United States, and in 1952, Erlacher established the correlation between the nucleogram and nuclear anatomy.[31, 94] Also in 1952, Cloward and Busaid described the indications and technique for lumbar discography.[16] Over the last four decades, indications, techniques, and treatment algorithms have improved significantly (Figures 4.8–4.10).

Lumbar discography is controversial and never fails to inspire heated debate. Antagonists of discography usually site a landmark study performed

Disc	vol.	L5-S1	L4-L5	L3-L4	L2-L3	L1-L2	vol.
Code		E (5)	D (4)	C (3)	B (2)	A (1)	
Discogram	0.5cc(1)						0.5cc(1)
Pain	1.0cc(2)						0cc(2)
Character	1.5cc(3)						1.5cc(3)
and	2.0cc(4)						2.0cc(4)
Intensity	2.5cc(5)						2.5cc(5)
	3.0cc(6)						3.0cc(6)
Final Volume							
Resistance		normal / increased / decreased	normal / increased / decreased	normal / increased / decreased	normal / increased / decreased	normal / increased / decreased	
Nucleogram							
End Point		firm / spongy / undefined	firm / spongy / undefined	firm / spongy / undefined	firm / spongy / undefined	firm / spongy / undefined	
Injection Side (L/R)							
IDET							
Misc.							
Versed Dose			Antibiotic				
Analgesic			Allergies				
Name			ID#		Date		

Discography Worksheet

Figure 4.8   Lumbar discogram worksheet. A properly performed discogram requires precise technique and careful documentation of findings.

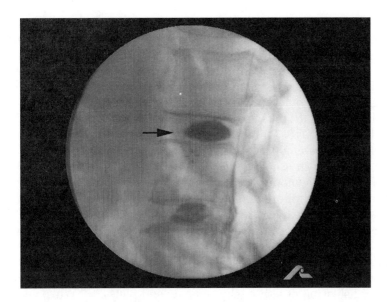

Figure 4.9   Normal lumbar discogram (arrow).

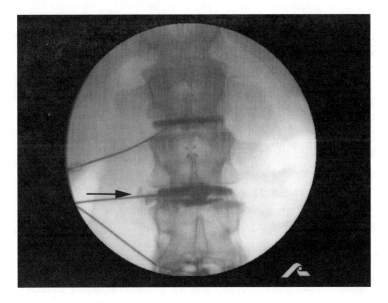

Figure 4.10   Abnormal lumbar discogram (arrow).

in 1968 by Earl Holt which demonstrated a 37% false-positive rate and concluded that discography was an unreliable tool.[52] Critics of the study point out several design flaws including poor imaging equipment used during the study, irritating contrast material, inadequate needle placement and not distinguishing a concordantly painful disc from a discordantly painful disc.[12, 82]

In 1990, Walsh et al. reevaluated Holt's data in seven patients with low back pain and ten asymptomatic volunteers using modern techniques and imaging tools.[90] He required that a discogram have both an abnormal morphology and a concordant pain response to be considered positive. In the asymptomatic group, none of the discograms were positive and in the symptomatic group 40% of the discs were considered positive. The significant factor in this study is the 0% false-positive rate of discography compared to the 37% false-positive rate found by Holt. Clearly, provocative testing for concordant pain is the single most important finding when determining whether a discogram is positive or negative. It is this factor that distinguishes discography from other anatomical imaging tools.

Even among supporters of discography and discographers themselves there remains debate over proper protocols and technique. Two areas of debate concern inadvertently making an asymptomatic disc appear symptomatic by overdistension or by performing a discogram adjacent to a symptomatic level without proper consideration. First, it has been determined that the normal lumbar disc accepts between 1 and 2 cc of volume and that overdistension of a disc may separate end plates.[4, 49] When end plates separate, other potentially painful structures may also be stretched causing pain thus confounding the interpretation of the discogram. As a result, many discographers use 2 cc as an arbitrary maximum volume to inject into a disc when attempting to provoke pain. Additional volume may be injected but a concordantly painful disc with a volume greater than that is considered "indeterminant." The obvious rationale in this approach is to be very clear about which discs are definitely symptomatic so that asymptomatic discs are not treated with destructive forms of surgery or other procedures.

Secondly, many discographers have noted that a disc adjacent to an exquisitely painful disc is often somewhat painful also. When this occurs, the discographer should inject the exquisitely painful disc with a 1/2 cc volume of 1% Lidocaine, wait 30 to 60 seconds and then reprovoke the adjacent, painful disc. What often happens is that the adjacent symptomatic disc becomes asymptomatic which probably indicates that there was some minor end plate motion of the exquisitely painful disc when injecting the adjacent level. By using these safeguards, the specificity of discography may remain high.

Discography has a limited but important role in the evaluation of the chronically painful spine. Other routine imaging techniques have supplanted discography for the evaluation of segmental anatomy but discography remains the only test that can stress each disc individually.

The indications for discography include: 1) determining which (if any) out of several abnormally appearing discs is symptomatic;[2, 68, 80] 2) as a component of an overall spinal injection diagnostic algorithm to ferret out the etiology of a patient's chronic pain;[4] 3) surgical decision making;[12, 17, 19, 44, 81] 4) evaluating a suspected lateral or recurrent disc;[14, 18, 19, 41, 43, 58, 59, 69] and 5) evaluating the integrity of a disc adjacent to a fusion.[14]

Patients selected for discography are interviewed for potential contraindications such as bleeding diathesis, systemic infection, unstable medical condition, and allergies to medications used in the procedure. Screening laboratory data on all patients include erythrocyte sedimentation rate, complete blood count, chemistry profile, and urinalysis. Patients over the age of 45 with a history positive for cardiac or pulmonary pathology, or a significant smoking history will also receive an electrocardiogram and a chest X-ray. Intravenous antibiotics are given to the patient to prophylax against infection immediately prior to and following the procedure and the patient is given a prescription for antibiotics upon discharge. Guyer has stated that due to the low incidence of discitis associated with discography, prophylactic antibiotics are optional.[46] Fraser has questioned this position, indicating that prior to the use of prophylactic antibiotics, the incidence of discitis was 2%. With the use of cephazolin for prophylaxis, discography was performed on a series of 3,250 patients with no known cases of discitis.[40]

Patient education is performed immediately prior to the procedure and includes the procedures indication, technique, time to completion, how to report the pain during the actual provocative process, the estimated time of pain following the procedure, and potential complications. The signs and symptoms of complication are reinforced to the patient and driver in the recovery room after the procedure and are given to them in written form upon discharge.

A typical screening lumbar discogram involves the lower three lumbar segments. Ideally, there should be a normal, or at least nonpainful, level out of these. If there is not, then an additional level or two should be done. If all levels are reported as painful then the patient's interpretation of pain is called into serious question since it is unclear as to what is considered pain. In addition, the patient's general tolerance for the procedure should be recorded as well since tolerance for somatic pain such as that caused by a discogram may have bearing on how well the patient may tolerate a significant insult like a fusion.

In trained hands the rate of complication is low. Potential complications include discitis, segmental nerve injury, dural puncture, aseptic meningitis, allergic reaction, and bleeding.[38, 42, 45, 67] These complications can be dramatically minimized by using sterile technique, screening out patients with a severe allergic history to contrast agents, using low ionic contrast agents, and making certain patients are off anti-inflammatory agents or other anticoagulants. Prophylactic antibiotics may further decrease the risk of infection.[37, 67] In addition, the reported incidence of discitis (0.05–4%) may be further minimized by utilizing a double needle technique.[38]

Discography remains controversial. The primary controversy involves the accuracy of the information supplied. When performed by experienced proceduralists, a high sensitivity and specificity can be maintained while minimizing complications.

4.8　Summary

Diagnostic spinal injections provide invaluable information that can significantly impact patient management decisions. A focused history and physical exam is important, however, a specific pain generator frequently is not identified. Imaging studies provide additional information, but the high rate of false positives can lead to questions regarding the source of pain.

The use of fluoroscopy is essential in order to ensure specific localization of needle placement. Fluoroscopy also eliminates the possibility of intravascular injection, reducing the overall risk of the injection procedures. Diagnostic information can be obtained from the patient's immediate response to local anesthetic and also from the delayed response to injected corticosteroids.

The techniques used for diagnostic injections have improved dramatically in the past few years. Further research is ongoing and is needed to refine current diagnostic strategies, and promote new diagnostic capabilities in the future.

4.9　References

1. Adams, M. Gradual disc prolapse, *Spine*, 10:524, 1985.
2. Antti-Poika, I. Clinical relevance of discography combined with CT scanning. A study of 100 patients, *J. Bone Joint Surg. [Br.]*, 72:480, 1990.
3. Aprill, C. The role of anatomically specific injections into the sacroiliac joint, presented at First Interdisciplinary World Congress on Low Back Pain and its Relation to the Sacroiliac Joint, San Diego, November 5, 1992.
4. Aprill, C. N. Diagnostic disc injection, *The Adult Spine: Principles and Practice*, in Frymore, J.W. ed., New York: Raven Press, 1991, 403.
5. Aprill, C. N. High intensity zone, *Br. J. Radiol.*, 65:361, 1992.
6. Bernard T. N. Jr., Cassidy, J. D. The sacroiliac joint syndrome pathophysiology, diagnosis, and management, in Frymoyer, J.W. ed., *The Adult Spine: Principles and Practice*, New York: Raven Press, 2107, 1991.
7. Boden, S. D., Davis, D. O., Dina, T. S. et al. Abnormal magnetic resource scans of the lumbar spine in asymptomatic subjects. A prospective investigation, *J. Bone. Joint, Surg. [Am.]*, 72:403, 1990.
8. Bogduk, N. Innervation of the lumbar spine, *Spine*, 8:286, 1983.
9. Bogduk, N. International spinal injection society guidelines for the performance of spinal injection Procedures. Part 1: Zygapophyseal joint blocks, *Clin. J. Pain.* December, 1997, 13(4):285–302.
10. Bogduk, N. Towmey, L. T., *Clinical Anatomy of the Lumbar Spine*, second ed., London: Churchill Livingstone, 1991.
11. Bonica, J. J., Buckley, F. P. Regional analgesic with local anesthetics, in *The Management of Pain*, Bonica, J. J., ed., Philadelphia: Lea & Febiger, 1990.
12. Brodsky, A. E. Lumbar discography: Its value in diagnosis and treatment of lumbar disc lesions, *Spine*, 4:110, 1979.
13. Brown, D. L. Lumbar sympathetic block, in *Atlas of Regional Anesthesia*, Philadelphia: W.B. Saunders 1992.

14. Butt, W. P. Discography: Some interesting cases, *J. Can. Ass. Radiol.*, XIV: 172, 1963.
15. Chapman, S. L., Brena, S. F. Learned helplessness and responses to nerve blocks in chronic low back pain patients, *Pain*, 14:355, 1982.
16. Cloward, R. B. Discography. Technique, indications, and evaluation of normal and abnormal intervertebral discs, *AJR: Am. J. Roentgenol.*, 68:552, 1952.
17. Colhoun, E. Provocation discography as a guide to planning operations on the spine, *J. Bone Joint. Surg. [Br.]*, 70:267, 1988.
18. Collins, H. R. An evaluation of cervical and lumbar discography, *Clin. Orthop.*, 107:133, 1975.
19. Collis, J. S. Lumbar discography: Analysis of 600 degenerative disks and diagnosis of degenerative disks disease, *JAMA*, 178:167, 1961.
20. Connally, G. H. Sanders, S. H. Predicting low back pain patients' response to lumbar sympathetic nerve blocks and interdisciplinary rehabilitation: The sole of pretreatment overt pain behavior and coping strategies, *Pain*, 44:139, 1991.
21. Crock, H. V. A reappraisal of intervertebral disc lesions, *Med. J. Aust.*, 1:983, 1970.
22. Derby, R. Point of view [letter], *Spine*, 19:1489, 1994.
23. Derby, R., Bogduk, N., Kine, G. Precision percutaneous blocking procedures for localizing spinal pain, part II, The lumbar neuraxial compartment, *Pain Digest*, 3:175, 1993.
24. Derby, R., Bogduk, N., Schwarzer, A. C. Precision percutaneous blocking procedures for localizing spinal pain, part I, The posterior lumbar compartment, *Pain Digest*, 3:89, 1993.
25. Dreyer, S., Dreyfuss, P., Cole, A. J. Zygapophyseal (facet) joint injections, intraarticular and medial branch block techniques, in Weinstein, S.M. ed., Injection techniques principle and practice, *Phys. Med. Rehabil. Clinics, N.A.*, Philadelphia: W. B. Saunders, 1996, 715.
26. Dreyer, S. J., Dreyfuss, P. H. Low back pain and the zygapophyseal (facet) joints, *Arch. Phys. Med. Rehabil.*, 77:290, 1996.
27. Dreyfuss, P., Cole, A. J., Pauza, K. Sacroiliac joint injection techniques. *Physical Med. Rehabil. Clinics, N.A.*, 6:785, 1995.
28. Dreyfuss, P., Lagattuta, F., Kaplansky, B. et al. Zygapophyseal joint injection techniques in the spinal axis, in Lennard, T.A. ed., *Physiatric Procedures in Clinical Practice*, Philadelphia: Hanley and Belfus, 1995, 206.
29. Dreyfuss, P., Michaelsen, M., Paucak, K. et al. The value of medical history and physical examination in diagnosing sacroiliac joint pain, *Spine* 1996, November 15; 21(22):2594–2602.
30. Dreyfuss, P., Schwarzer, A. C., Lau, P. et al. Specificity of lumbar medial branch and L5 dorsal ramus blocks, *Spine* (22)8:895–902.
31. Erlacker, P. R. Nucleography, *J. Bone Joint Surg. [Br.]*, 34:204, 1952.
32. Farfan, H. F. Lumbar intervertebral disc degeneration. The influence of geometrical features on the pattern of disc degeneration — a post mortem study, *J. Bone Joint Surg. [Am.]*, 54:492, 1972.
33. Farfan, H. F. The effects of torsion on the lumbar intervertebral joints: The role of torsion on disc degeneration, *J. Bone Joint Surg. [Am.]*, 52:468, 1970.
34. Fortin, J. Sacroiliac joint injection and arthrography with imaging correlation, *Physiatric Procedures in Clinical Practice*, Lennard, T., Ed., Philadelphia: Hanley & Belfus, 1995.

35. Fortin, J. D., Dwyer, A., Aprill, C. et al. Sacroiliac joint pain referral patterns, part II: Clinical evaluation, *Spine*, 19:1483, 1994.
36. Fortin, J. D., Dwyer, A., West, S. et al. Sacroiliac joint pain referral patterns upon application of a new injection/arthrography technique, part I: Asymptomatic volunteers, *Spine*, 19:1475, 1994.
37. Fortin, J. D., Tolahin, R. Sacroiliac arthrograms and postarthrography CT, *Arch. Phys. Med. Rehabil.*, 74:1259, 1993.
38. Fraser, R. D. Discitis after discography, *J. Bone Joint Surg. [Br.]*, 69:26, 1969.
39. Fraser, R. D. Iatrogenic discitis: The role of intravenous antibiotics in prevention and treatment, *Spine*, 14:1025, 1989.
40. Fraser, R. D. Letter, *Spine* 21(10):1274–1278, 1996.
41. Fries, J. W. Computed tomography of herniated and extruded nucleus pulposus, *J. Comput. Assist. Tomogr.*, 6:874, 1972.
42. Gardner, W. J. X-ray visualization of the intervertebral disc: With a consideration of the morbidity of disc puncture, *Arch. Surg.*, 64:355, 1952.
43. Godersky, J. C. Extreme lateral disc herniation: Diagnosis by computed tomographic scanning, *Neurosurgery*, 14:1974.
44. Gresham, J. L. Evaluation of the lumbar spine by diskography and its use in selection of the proper treatment of the herniated disk syndrome, *Clin. Orthop.*, 67:29, 1969.
45. Guyer, R. D. Discitis after discography *Spine*, 13:1352, 1988.
46. Guyer, R. D., Ohnmeiss, D. D. Contemporary concepts in spine care lumbar discography: Position statement from the north american spine society diagnostic and therapeutic committee. *Spine* (20)18:2048–2059, 1995.
47. Hauseisen, D. C., Smith, B. S., Myers, S. R. et al. The diagnostic accuracy of spinal nerve injection studies: their role in the evaluation of recurrent sciatica, *Clin. Orthop.*, 198:179, 1985.
48. Haynesworth, R. F., Noe, C. E., Fassy, L. R. Intralymphatic injection: Another complication of lumbar sympathetic block, *Anesth.*, 80:460, 1994.
49. Heggeness, M. Discography causes end plate deflection, *Spine*, 18:1050, 1993.
50. Herron, L. D. Selective nerve root block in patient selection for lumbar surgery; Surgical results, *J. Spinal Disorders*, 2:75, 1989.
51. Hirsch, C. Attempt to diagnose the level of disc lesion by puncture. *Acta. Orthop. Scand.*, 18:131, 1948.
52. Holt, E. P. The question of lumbar discography, *J. Bone Joint Surg. [Am.]*, 50:720, 1968.
53. Ikeda, R. Innervation of the sacroiliac joint. Macroscopical and histological studies. *Nippon Ika Daigaku Zasshi* October 1991 58(5):587–96.
54. Jaffray, D. Isolated intervertebral disc resorption. A source of mechanical and inflammatory back pain? *Spine*, 11:397, 1986.
55. Jaovisidha, S., Ryu, K. N., De Maeseneer et al. Ventral sacroiliac ligament anatomic and pathologic considerations, *Invest. Radiology* 1996 August, 31(8):532–41.
56. Kaplan, M., Dreyfuss, P., Halbrook, B. et al. The ability of lumbar medial branch blocks to anesthetize the zygapophysial joint, *Spine* (23)17:1847–1852.
57. Kirkald-Willis, W. H. Pathology and pathogenesis of lumbar spondylosis and stenosis, *Spine*, 3:319, 1978.
58. Kornberg, M. Extreme lateral lumbar disc herniation, *Spine*, 12:586, 1987.
59. Kurobane, Y. Extraforaminal disc herniation, *Spine*, 11:260, 1987.

60. Lindblom, K. Diagnostic puncture of the intervertebral disc in sciatica, *Acta. Orthop. Scand.*, 17:231, 1948.
61. Lord, S. M., Barnsley, L., Bogduk, N., The utility of comparative local anesthetic blocks versus placebo-controlled blocks for the diagnosis of cervical zygapophysial joint pain, *Clin. J. of Pain*, 11:208–213, 1995.
62. Luschka, H. *Die Halbgelenke des Menschlichen Korpers.* Berlin: G Rheimers, 1858.
63. Maigne, J. Y., Aivaliklis, A., Pfefer, F. Results of sacroiliac joint double block and value of sacroiliac pain provocation tests in 54 patients with low back pain, August, *Spine* August, 1996 15; 21(16):1889–92.
64. McCarron, R. F. The inflammatory effects of nucleus pulposus: A possible element in the pathogenesis of low back pain, *Spine*, 12:760, 1987.
65. Mixter, W. J. Rupture of the intervertebral disc with involvement of the spinal canal, *N. Engl. J. Med.*, 211:157, 1934.
66. Mooney, V., Robertson, J. Facet joint syndrome, *Clin. Ortho.*, 115:149, 1976.
67. Osti, O. L. Discitis after discography. The role of prophylactic antibiotics, *J. Bone Joint Surg.*, 72:271, 1990.
68. Patton, J. T. Discography in assessment of lumbar disc disease, *Ann. Rheum. Dis.*, 34:466, 1975.
69. Preacher, W. G. The roentgen diagnosis of herniated disk with particular reference to discography (nucleography), *AJR: Am. J. Roentgenol.*, 76:290, 1956.
70. Saal, J. High levels of inflammatory phospholipase A2 in lumbar disc herniations. *Spine*, 15:674, 1990.
71. Saal, J. Nonoperative treatment of herniated lumbar intervertebral disc with radiculopathy, *Spine*, 14:431, 1989.
72. Saal, J. The natural history of lumbar intervertebral disc extrusions treated conservatively, *Spine*, 15:1990.
73. Schmorl, G. Uber Knorpelknoten an der Hinterflache der Werbelbandscheiben, *Fortsch. Rontgenstr.*, 40:629, 1929.
74. Schwarzer, A. C., Aprill, C. N., Bogduk, N. The sacroiliac joint in chronic low back pain, *Spine*, 20:31, 1995.
75. Schwarzer, A. C., Aprill, C. N., Derby, R. et al. The relative contributions of the disc and zygapophyseal joint in chronic LBP, *Spine*, 19:801, 1994.
76. Schwarzer, A. C., Aprill, C. N., Fortin, J. et al. The clinical features of patients with pain stemming from the lumbar zygapophyseal joints: Is the lumbar facet syndrome a clinical entity?, *Spine*, 19:1132, 1994.
77. Schwarzer, A. C., Derby, R., Aprill, C. N. et al. The value of the provocation response in lumbar zygapophyseal joint injections, *Clin. J. Pain*, 10:309, 1994.
78. Schwarzer, A. C., Wang, S., Bogduk, N. et al. Prevalence and clinical features of lumbar zygapophyseal joint pain: A study in an Australian population with chronic low back pain, *Ann. Rheum. Dis.*, 54:100, 1995.
79. Schwarzer, A. C., Wang, S., O'Driscoll, D. et al. The ability to computed tomography to identify a painful zygapophyseal joint in patients with chronic low back pain, *Spine*, 20:907, 1995.
80. Simmons, E. H. Discography: Localization of symptomatic levels, *J. Bone Joint Surg. [Br.]*, 57:261, 1975.
81. Simmons, E. H. An evaluation of discography in the localization of symptomatic levels in discogenic disease of the spine, *Clin. Orthop. Rel. Res.*, 108:57, 1975.
82. Simmons, J. W., A reassessment of Holt's data on the question of lumbar discography, *Clin. Orthop. Rel. Res.*, 237:120, 1988.

83. Slipman, C. W. Diagnostic nerve root blocks, in *Neural Blockade in Clinical Anesthesia and Management of Pain. second edition.* Cousins, M. J., Bridenbaugh, P. O., ed., Philadelphia: Lippincott; 253–360, 1988.

84. Slipman, C. W., Sterenfeld, E. B., Chou, L. H. et al. The predictive value of provacative sacroiliac joint stress maneuvers in the diagnosis of sacroiliac joint syndrome, *Arch. PM&R* March, 1998, 79:288–292.

85. Solonen, K. A. The sacroiliac joint in light of anatomical, roentgenological, and clinical studies, *Acta. Orthop. Scand.,* 27:1, 1957.

86. Sprague, R. S., Ramamurthy, S. Identification of the anterior psoas sheath as a landmark for lumbar sympathetic block, *Reg. Anesth.,* 15:253, 1990.

87. Stanley, D., McLoren, M. I., Evinton, H. A. et al. A prospective study of nerve root infiltration in the diagnosis of sciatica: A comparison with radiculopathy, computed tomography and operative findings, *Spine,* 15:540, 1990.

88. Steindler, A. Differential diagnosis of pain in the low back: Allocation of the source of pain by procaine hydrochloride method, *JAMA,* 110:106, 1938.

89. Umeda, S., Arani, T., Hatano, Y. et al. Cadaveric anatomic analysis of the best site for chemical lumbar sympathectomy, *Anesth. Analg.,* 66:643, 1987.

90. Walsh, T. R. Lumbar discography in normal subjects, *J. Bone Joint Surg. [Am.],* 72:1081, 1990.

91. Weber, H. Lumbar disc herniation: A controlled prospective study with 10 years of observation, *Spine,* 8:131, 1983.

92. Weisel, S. W., Tsourmas, N., Feffer, H. L. et al. A study of computer-assisted tomography, part I, The incidence of positive CT scans on asymptomatic patients, *Spine,* 9:549, 1984.

93. Windsor, R. E., Lester, J. P., Dreyer, S. J., Cervicothoracic and lumbar sympathetic blockade, *Physiatric Procedures in Clinical Practice,* Lennard, T., Ed., Philadelphia: Hanley & Belfus, 1995.

94. Wise, R. E., X-ray visualization of the intervertebral disc, *Clev. Clinic Q.,* 18:127, 1990.

95. Woodward, J. L., Herring, S. A., Windsor, R. E. et al. Epidural procedures in spine pain management, in *Physiatric Procedures in Clinical Practice,* Lennard, T. A., ed., Philadelphia: Hanley & Belfus, Inc., 1995.

96. Wulf, H., Gleim, M., Schele, H. Plasma concentrations of bupivacaine after lumbar sympathetic block, *Anesth. Analg.,* 79:918, 1994.

chapter five

The Functional Capacity Evaluation

Boris Terebuh, M.D.
Nathan Notter, P.T.

5.1 Overview

The functional capacity evaluation (FCE) is a tool that strives to generate objective data which more comprehensively defines an individual's maximum physical ability. A series of test activities is administered to measure whether an individual has the ability to meet a particular level of function.[6] There are three major contexts in which the utilization of an FCE is considered: 1) industrial medicine; 2) litigation, product liability, and personal injury; and 3) other injury or disability compensation systems.[18] The purpose of this chapter is to explore the role of the FCE in industrial medicine and specifically in the context of low back pain (LBP) which results from occupational injury.

5.2 Protocols

In the past two decades FCE protocols have become more numerous.[22–31] FCEs are now more sought after by employers and insurers who have grown more reliant upon them.[6] There exists the perception that the data generated from an FCE is more objective and therefore more helpful in making decisions regarding injured workers and return-to-work issues. FCE protocols can vary significantly in their design and administration. The majority can be completed in a few hours but one particular protocol advocates a two-day testing period.[26] Beyond the assertions of the protocol originators, there is no objective data to justify any given length of FCE testing.

FCEs can be broadly categorized as job-specific or nonjob-specific. A job-specific FCE measures only the critical work demands of a specific job requirement. The critical work demands are those aspects of the injured worker's (IW) job which will affect the injured body part to the greatest degree and which will prevent the worker from returning to work or cause a reinjury after return to work.[4] An accurate job description is essential for an evaluator to properly test critical work demands. Job-specific FCE protocols are the shortest in length of administration and lowest in cost. A nonjob-specific FCE measures a wide range of activities including, at times, entire body function. Often all twenty physical demands of work described by the Dictionary of Occupational Titles (DOT) are tested.[19] Such FCE protocols are more lengthy and more costly.

5.3　Validity

Although heavy lifting is a known risk factor in work-related back injuries, performing lifting tasks alone in a limited job-specific FCE is usually not sufficient to define work tolerance in the context of work related injuries. In some circumstances, IWs continue to report pain and dysfunction despite the fact that all appropriate diagnostic and therapeutic options have been pursued. Low back pain, whether real, imagined, or embellished is impossible to quantify and integrity of effort is even more difficult to gauge. An added advantage of a nonjob-specific FCE is that additional parameters are monitored which provide the opportunity to measure consistency of effort. Such parameters are referred to as validity criteria. A nonjob-specific FCE often incorporates validity criteria which can be interspersed throughout the evaluation to test the sincerity of effort put forth by the IW. The purpose of validity criteria is to help determine if the FCE data represents maximal effort and to help determine if the FCE data should be used to determine the IW's current work ability.[4] This is crucial information for the clinician to ensure that appropriate conclusions are drawn regarding the IW's true functional capacity. An inconsistent effort is used as grounds to invalidate the IW's performance on the FCE.

Fluctuations of greater than 15% between successive repetitions of static (isometric) lifting activities suggest inconsistency in effort.[4] A five-position hand grip test should produce a modified bell-shaped curve to represent maximum effort.[16] One should expect successive trials of range of motion of the trunk to fall within 10% or 5 degrees when measuring with an inclinometer. Anything greater suggests a lack of consistency of effort.[3] The Borg Rating of Perceived Exertion (RPE) heart rate difference multiplies the reported Borg RPE[5] value times 10 and then subtracts the actual heart rate at the time of the activity. If the resultant value ranges between 20 to 50 units, the difference can be explained based on a physiologic pain response. A resultant value greater than 50 suggests submaximal effort or symptom magnification. In order to measure this parameter, heart rate monitoring equipment is necessary. Other parameters used to test validity include: cogwheel (ratchety) muscle release on strength testing,[20] the presence of Waddell's nonorganic signs,[21] and the Somatic Amplification Rating Scale.[7]

The FCE data should be considered valid regardless of the IW's performance because it represents the degree of effort that was exerted.[4] To proclaim the FCE as invalid implies that the FCE itself is flawed. It is more accurate to state that the IW's performance was invalid.

Validity of the FCE result is considered to resolve whether or not the data can or should be used to determine the IW's accurate return-to-work ability.[4] Despite the common practice of declaring an IW's performance invalid based on inconsistent isometric testing, no literature has definitively established that inconsistent performance on isometric testing is associated with inconsistent and submaximal performance during dynamic activities.[9] The assumption remains, however, that inconsistent isometric performance raises enough suspicion to question the sincerity of effort in the remainder of the FCE.

An FCE is usually administered by an occupational therapist or a physical therapist. Other professionals who also administer FCEs include: specifically trained vocational evaluators, nurses, exercise physiologists, and kinesiologists. Six factors potentially limit an IW's ability to lift: symptoms, leg strength, trunk strength, arm strength, body mechanics, and motivation.[4] Material handling (dynamic lifting) testing is terminated if there is an increase in pain symptoms, failure to complete an activity due to lack of strength, failure to maintain proper body mechanics, effort level appears to be maximized, or if the IW requests that testing be terminated. The evaluator should always document the reason for terminating an activity. It is obviously essential for the FCE administrator to be knowledgeable regarding proper body mechanics. Subjectivity is therefore introduced into the FCE process on two levels. The IW can terminate an activity with a subjective report of excessive pain and the administrator of the FCE can terminate an activity if the lifting technique is deemed unsafe.

5.4　Indications

Before an IW can be considered for an FCE all diagnostic evaluations and therapeutic interventions for the etiology of LBP should be complete. A possible exception to this principle is when an FCE is undertaken to establish the least restrictive, yet safe, temporary work parameters for an IW who is in the process of undergoing treatment for a work injury. The population in which a FCE is usually considered is one in which there is residual LBP and or physical dysfunction even after all diagnostic and therapeutic options have been pursued. The presence of pain or dysfunction notwithstanding, an IW's condition must be medically stable prior to consideration of an FCE. An inappropriately or incompletely treated medical condition, an exaggerated pain experience, or excessive deconditioning are all factors which can adversely effect performance by an IW on an FCE. Guidelines established by the American Physical Therapy Association[17] are followed to set criteria for the performance testing battery. The guidelines have established a hierarchy of criteria which in descending order of significance include: safety, reliability, validity, practicality, and utility. All five criteria must be met by the performance test before it is administered to the IW.

It is beyond the scope of this chapter to expound in detail on each of the numerous established FCE protocols in existence, but some of the common protocols are cited in the references for further independent review.[22-31] Rather, the major components of an FCE will be listed. These major components include: 1) record review, 2) self-administered questionnaire, 3) interview, 4) musculoskeletal evaluation, 5) physiological measures, 6) functional measures, and 7) comparison of testing with job requirements.[6] Parts 1–4 and 7 are self-explanatory and the role of Parts 1–4 are primarily important to identify any particular contraindications to performing specific activities in a given FCE. Parts 5 and 6 are elaborated upon below.

5.5   Measurements

Physiologic measures deal primarily with muscular and cardiovascular endurance. Continuous heart rate monitoring is necessary to adequately measure these parameters. Functional measures include isometric (static) activities and dynamic activities. Isometric activities include the hand dynamometer, the pinch gauge, and the static strength gauge, which can be adjusted to accommodate various lifting postures (Figure 5.1). Isometric tests correlate poorly with performance on dynamic functional tasks.[8] On the other hand, free dynamic lifting protocols have been criticized for inadequate anatomic stabilization, subjectivity involved when the IW declares the end point to lifting activities, and lack of control for speed and acceleration variables.[2, 11, 12] Dynamic lifting activities such as material handling are most often tested using containers of various dimensions into which weight is placed (Figure 5.2). In some protocols the weight of a one-time maximum lift for a given lifting posture[24] is compared to normative data[13, 14, 15] to extrapolate recommended weights for occasional and frequent lifting. This process is repeated for each lifting posture. Other protocols establish the weight for frequent lifting as a percentage of the weight that can be lifted safely on an occasional basis.[27] Some feel that the use of formulas and percentages to extrapolate lifting limits introduces an unacceptable degree of error to the process.[6]

The terms occasional, frequent, and constant are physical demand levels which have been defined by the *Dictionary of Occupational Titles*.[19] An activity occurring on an occasional basis can involve 0 to 33% of the daily work shift. In terms of repetitions, an occasional activity may involve 1 to 32 repetitions per work shift. Frequent activities involve 34 to 66% of the work shift or 33 to 200 repetitions. Constant activities occupy 67 to 100% of the work shift or greater than 200 repetitions in that time period. Sedentary, light, medium, heavy, and very heavy work designations also exist and lifting limits for each category vary depending on the physical demand level in each category (Table 5.1).

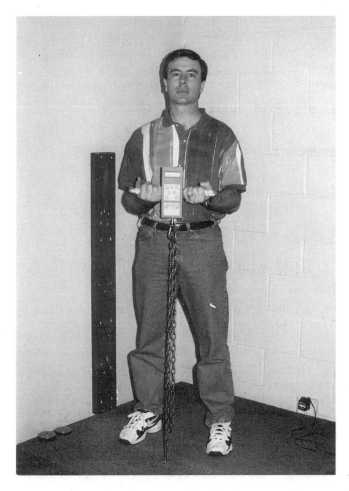

Figure 5.1 Isometric lifting can be measured with a static strength gauge. The chain length can be adjusted to accommodate various lifting positions.

Table 5.1

Physical Demand Level	Occasional 0–33% of work time 1–32 reps	Frequent 34–66% of work time 33–200 reps	Constant 67–100% of work time >200 reps
Sedentary	10 lbs	Negligible	Negligible
Light	20 lbs	10 lbs	Negligible
Medium	50 lbs	20 lbs	10 lbs
Heavy	100 lbs	50 lbs	20 lbs
Very Heavy	>100 lbs	>50 lbs	>20 lbs

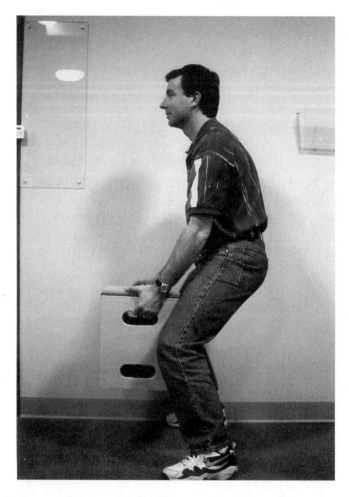

Figure 5.2   Dynamic lifting is tested with material handling. The wooden box can be opened to accommodate varying amounts of weight. Multiple lifting positions can be tested with material handling. Here the subject is demonstrating a floor to waist lift.

A sample hybrid FCE report, which is an amalgam of multiple protocols, is included below and serves as an example of how results may appear in report format.

5.5.1   A Hybrid Functional Capacity Evaluation Report

PATIENT: John Doe

HISTORY: Reported by patient
Patient is a 32-year-old right-hand-dominant male who initially injured his low back while bending and lifting plywood. He reported his injury to his supervisor and was referred to the company physician where he was

diagnosed with a low back strain. Physical therapy did not resolve his pain symptoms and he was subsequently referred to a specialist. Diagnostic tests performed included an EMG (normal) and an MRI of the lumbosacral spine (normal). Patient returned to work for approximately six weeks despite continued low back pain.

PAST MEDICAL HISTORY
Lumbar fusion at L4-L5, 1996

CURRENT COMPLAINTS
Patient states that he has pain in his low back without radiation into the lower limbs. He experiences increased symptoms with bending, twisting, sitting in one position for 5–10 minutes, standing in one position for 30–40 minutes, and with walking for 5–10 minutes. His symptoms are relieved by lying down.

JOB DESCRIPTION: Reported by Patient
Patient is currently employed as a general laborer which requires him to lift up to 50 lbs. from floor to shoulder level constantly during his work shift. He works indoors for eight-hour shifts, five days per week, with optional over-time. Patient sits rarely, stands constantly, walks constantly, stair climbs occasionally, bends frequently, reaches overhead frequently, squats frequently, kneels frequently, pivot twists frequently, reaches forward occasionally, pushes occasionally, pulls occasionally, repetitive reaches frequently, writes occasionally, stacks objects frequently, performs fine motor skills frequently, and performs forearm and wrist movements frequently during his work shift. He may be required to drive a forklift and at times use a hammer.

Rarely	Less than 5% of an eight-hour work shift
Occasionally	0–33% of an eight-hour work shift
Frequently	34–66% of an eight-hour work shift
Constantly	67–100% of an eight-hour work shift

CLINICAL FINDINGS
Observation: Patient is deconditioned.
Pain Rating: Patient rates his low back pain a 5/10 prior to beginning the functional capacity evaluation with 0 representing no pain and 10 indicating pain of sufficient intensity to seek emergency medical care.
Heart Rate: Patient presents with a resting heart rate of 65 beats per minute as measured by a pulsar monitor with a watch.
Blood Pressure: Patient's blood pressure is 120/80.
Posture: Patient's posture is within functional limits.
Gait: Patient presents with a normal tandem gait.
Palpation: Patient complains of pain with palpation to the bilateral piriformis muscles, bilateral lumbar paraspinal muscles, as well as over the L3, L4, L5, and S1 vertebral levels.

Lumbar Active Range of Motion:

Flexion:	50%
Extension:	75%
Sidebend Right:	75%
Sidebend Left:	75%
Rotation Right:	75%
Rotation Left:	75%

Note: Patient complains of increased low back pain at the end of range of motion for all lumbar movements tested above.

Muscle Strength:

Upper Abdominals	4/5
Lower Abdominals	4 − /5
Back Extensors	4 − /5

Bilateral Lower Limb Active Range of Motion: Within normal limits in his hips, knees, and ankles.

Bilateral Lower Limb Muscle Strength:

Movement	Right	Left
Hip Flexion	5/5	4+/5
Extension	5/5	4+/5
Abduction	5/5	4+/5
Adduction	5/5	4+/5
Knee Flexion	5/5	4+/5
Knee Extension	5/5	4+/5
Ankle Dorsiflexion	5/5	5/5
Ankle Plantar Flexion	5/5	5/5

Note: Patient had no subjective complaints of increased pain present in the low back during lower limb strength testing.

Special Test:
Waddell's Test: Negative for all Waddell's tests performed during the functional capacity evaluation.

5.5.2 Functional Capacity Evaluation

REPETITIVE MOVEMENT TEST:
Gait Pattern: Patient presents with a normal tandem gait.
Bending × 1: Patient demonstrated approximately 50% range of motion with bending forward for one repetition. Patient's velocity was normal. He complained of increased low back pain at the end range of motion while bending forward for one repetition.
Bending × 10: Patient has 50% range of motion present while bending forward during 10 repetitions with complaints of marked increase in low back pain. Patient's heart rate increased from 60 beats per minute to 85 beats per minute while bending forward for 10 repetitions.

Fast Bending × 10: Not performed due to patient's subjective complaints of marked increased pain present in the low back with bending forward. Movement ability was determined to be *never* for this activity. Movement correlated with patient's pain.

Reaching × 1: Patient is able to reach overhead with normal range of motion, velocity, and rhythm. Patient had no complaints of increased low back pain while reaching overhead for one repetition.

Reaching × 10: Patient again demonstrated normal range of motion, velocity, and rhythm. Patient had no complaints of increased low back pain.

Fast Reaching × 10: Repetitions were completed in seven seconds (normal is less than eight seconds). Patient had no increase in low back pain while reaching overhead for 10 fast repetitions. Movement ability was determined to be *frequent* for this activity. Movement did not correlate with patient's pain.

Squatting × 1: Patient has normal range of motion, velocity, and rhythm during squatting for one repetition. Patient had no subjective complaints of increased low back pain while squatting for one repetition.

Squatting × 10: Patient had normal range of motion, velocity, and rhythm while squatting for 10 repetitions. Patient had no subjective complaints of increased low back pain. Patient complained of being tired and demonstrated mild to minimum fatigue while squatting for 10 repetitions.

Squatting × 10-Second Set: Patient demonstrated moderate fatigue with normal range of motion and reduced velocity. Patient did complain of increased low back pain while squatting for a second set of 10 repetitions. Movement ability was determined to be *occasional* for this activity. Movement did not correlate with patient's pain.

NONMATERIAL HANDLING SKILLS:

Sitting: Patient was able to sit during the functional capacity evaluation for approximately 30 minutes in one position continuously prior to having to move due to subjective complaints of increased pain. This would extrapolate to *occasional* sitting ability.

Stand/Walk: During the functional capacity evaluation, patient was able to perform standing and walking activities for approximately 60 minutes continuously prior to requesting to sit down due to subjective complaints of feeling tired and increased low back pain. This would extrapolate to *frequent* standing and walking ability.

Stair Climbing: Patient is able to climb up and down stairs *frequently.*

FIVE-POSITION GRIP TEST: The Five-Position Grip Test is used to determine the reliability of the subject's efforts. Test scores should form a bell curve from Position I through V.

HAND	I	II	III	IV	V
Left	140#	145#	158#	150#	140#
Right	135#	148#	160#	151#	132#

Note: Bilateral hands demonstrate a bell curve for the Five-Position Grip Test which indicates that the patient gave a valid effort during this portion of the test.

STATIC GRIP AND PINCH STRENGTH TESTING

TEST	AVERAGE	C.V.	% RANK
Right Position 2 Grip	165#	5.8%	89th
Left Position 2 Grip	158.2#	5%	90th
Right Tip Pinch	20.0#	9.4%	64th
Left Tip Pinch	18.4#	1.8%	52nd
Right Palmer Pinch	23#	5.9%	42nd
Left Palmer Pinch	21#	2.8%	3rd
Right Key Pinch	20#	6.8%	63rd
Left Key Pinch	19.5#	5%	56th

STATIC STRENGTH TESTING

TEST	AVERAGE	C.V.	% RANK
Arm Lift	85.5#	8.9%	55th
High Near Lift	122#	12.4%	51st
High Far Lift	58#	11.2%	66th
Torso Lift	N/A	N/A	N/A
Leg Lift	112#	20.2%	11th
Push	116#	18.2%	52nd
Pull	152#	12.4%	39th

Note: Patient complained of increased low back pain with performance of the leg lift and push portions of the static strength testing. The coefficient of variation (C.V.) exceeded 15% for these two tests indicating that he did not produce a valid effort during these portions of the functional capacity evaluation. The patient was unable to assume the proper position for the torso lift due to a subjective report of increased low back pain.

Critical Job Demands	Physical Work Strengths	Job Match
Use of Tools — Occasionally	Right Hand Grip 165#	Yes
	Left Hand Grip 158#	Yes
Floor — Waist Lift (1–50#) frequently	Floor — Waist Lift (1–40#) — occasionally	No
Front Carry Boxes (1–50#) frequently	30-foot Front Carry 50# — frequently	Yes
Waist-Shoulder Lift (1–50#) frequently	Waist — Shoulder Lift 50# frequently	Yes
Stand — constantly	Stand — frequently	No
Walk — constantly	Walk — frequently	No
Stair Climb — occasionally	Stair Climb — occasionally	Yes
Forward Bend — frequently	Forward Bend — unable	No
Reach Overhead — frequently	Reach Overhead — frequently	Yes
Push/Pull — occasionally	Push/Pull — occasionally	Yes
Squat — frequently	Squat — occasionally	No

ASSESSMENT AND RECOMMENDATIONS

1. Patient's physical abilities do match some portions of the job description for his position as a general laborer. Mismatches were the

result of the patient's subjective report of increased pain with various activities.

2. Patient's heart rate and blood pressure increased appropriately during FCE testing.

3. Work modifications which may be helpful include: substituting waist to shoulder lifting in place of floor to waist lifting because the former did not increase low back pain symptoms; changing positions between sitting, standing, and walking to decrease low back pain symptoms.

5.6 Limitations

The authors of this chapter do not endorse one particular FCE protocol over any of the others. The selection of an FCE protocol is usually dictated by what type of information is desired (job-specific or nonjob-specific). There is also a regional bias for various FCE protocols which may be most influenced by differences in workers compensation laws from state to state. Some states require vocational retraining and placement of an IW in a new job after a work-related injury. A nonjob-specific FCE would therefore be of more utility. In other states permanent work restrictions are generated if the IW cannot return to the original job but retraining or placement is not pursued.

Questions remain regarding the validity of entire FCE protocols with respect to predicting return-to-work issues. Few studies exist in the literature which address this question. Little published peer-reviewed research has documented the reliability and validity of FCE protocols[10] and few[28, 29] have demonstrated intra- and interrater reliability under the scrutiny of peer review. Another concern is that performance on an FCE does not predict accurately functional performance over a typical eight-hour work shift.[1] For this reason a two-day testing period for an FCE has been advocated[26] to better account for fatigue, but no peer-reviewed literature has been published to support this position.

Most FCE protocols are enterprises that require prospective test administrators to participate in a training course which involves payment of tuition to the protocol originators. Other FCE protocols have developed trademarked equipment with which the testing is performed[22] (Figure 5.3). The originators of the majority of established FCEs have not subjected their protocols to the scrutiny of peer review to determine if they are reliable or valid methods of measuring maximum physical function.

5.7 Summary

The FCE attempts to make more objective the process by which work limitations are determined. Ultimately subjectivity is introduced into the process as the determination of what constitutes a safe lifting technique is left to the interpretation of the test administrator and the IW can terminate an activity with subjective reports of pain. FCE protocols have many other potential

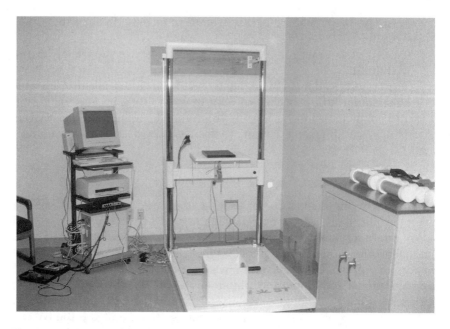

Figure 5.3 An example of commercially available computerized FCE equipment which also can monitor heart rate.

pitfalls: static lifting activities do not correlate well with dynamic lifting activities, simulated work approximates but is not identical to the real work environment, and the data generated from an FCE has not been proven to be predictive of injury potential when generalized to an eight-hour work shift. The use of isometric validity criteria to determine whether or not an IW's dynamic performance is valid is a practice that can also be questioned because no correlation has been proven in the literature. Although many questions remain regarding the validity, predictive value, and interrater reliability of the various FCE protocols, they remain widely used in the process of defining functional limitations, especially in the context of work-related low back pain. Further prospective research is certainly necessary to determine if any particular FCE protocol has a positive predictive value in determining return-to-work status.

The FCE process is certainly not immune from the threat of litigation. Malpractice settlements against physicians have been awarded to IWs who claimed that they sustained injury while undergoing an FCE ordered by the physician. This is an unfortunate reality in the sometimes adversarial system of the workers compensation programs from state to state. It is uncertain how these precedent-setting cases will affect the future use of the FCE in the context of work-related LBP. As with any other form of diagnostic or therapeutic intervention being considered for an IW, thought should be given to the pros, cons, and limitations of a functional capacity evaluation before one is ordered.

5.8 References

1. Abdel-Moty, E., Fishbain, D., Khalil, T. et al. Functional capacity and residual functional capacity and their utility in measuring work capacity, *Clin. J. of Pain* 9:168–173, 1993.
2. Alpert, J., Matheson, L., Beam, W. et al. The reliability and validity of two new tests of maximum lifting capacity, *J. of Occup. Rehabil.* 1:13–29, 1991.
3. *American Medical Association: Guides to the Evaluation of Permanent Impairment.* Chicago: AMA, 4th ed., 1993.
4. Blankenship, K. L. *Industrial Rehabilitation: A Seminar Syllabus.* Macon, GA: American Therapeutics, 1990.
5. Borg, G. A. V. Psychophysical basis of perceived exertion, *Med. Sci. Sports. Exercise.* 14:377–381, 1982.
6. King, P., Tuckwell, N., Barrett, T. A critical review of functional capacity evaluations, *Phys. Ther.* 78(8):852–866, 1998.
7. Korbon, G. A., DeGood, D. E., Schroeder, M. et al. The development of the somatic amplification rating scale for low back pain, *Spine* 12:787–791, 1987.
8. Kroemer, K. An isoinertial technique to assess individual lifting capacity. *Hum. Factors* 25:493–506, 1983.
9. Lechner, D. E., Roth, D., Straaton, K. Functional capacity evaluation in work disability, *Work* 1:37–47, 1991.
10. Lechner, D. E., Jackson, J. R., Roth, D. L. et al. Reliability and validity of a newly developed test of physical work performance, *J. of Occup. Med.* 36:997–1004, 1994.
11. Matheson, L. N. Evaluation of lifting and lowering capacity, *Vocational Evaluation and Work Adjustment Bull.* Fall 107–111, 1986.
12. Mital, A., A psychophysical approach in manual lifting: A verification study. *Hum. Factors* 25:485–491, 1983.
13. *NIOSH — Work Practices Guide for Manual Lifting.* U.S. Department of Health and Human Services, Pub. No. 81–122, CDC, Cincinnati, OH, 1981.
14. Snook, S. H., Irvine, H., Bass, S. F. Maximum Weight and Workloads Acceptable to Male Industrial Workers. *Amer. Ind. Hyg. Assoc. J.* 3:579, 1970.
15. Snook, S. H. The design of manual handling tasks. *Ergonomics* 21:963–985, 1978.
16. Stokes, H. M. The seriously injured hand: Weakness of grip. *J. of Occup. Med.* 25:683–684, 1983.
17. Task force on standards for measurement in physical therapy: Standards for tests and measurements in physical therapy practice. *Phys. Ther.* 71(8):589–622, 1991.
18. Tramposh, A. K. The functional capacity evaluation: Measuring maximal work abilities. *Occup. Med.: State of the Art Rev.* 7(1):113–124, 1992.
19. *U.S. Department of Labor, Employment, and Training Administration: Revised Dictionary of Occupational Titles.* vol. I, vol. II. Fourth edition Washington, DC: U.S. Government Printing Office, 1991.
20. Waddell, G., McCulloch, J. A., Kummel, E. et al. Nonorganic physical signs in low back pain. *Spine* 5:117–125, 1980.
21. Waddell, G., Main, C. J., Morris, E. W. et al. Chronic low back pain, psychologic distress and illness behavior. *Spine* 9:209–213, 1984.

Functional Capacity Evaluation Protocols

22. *ARCON Users' Guide.* Williamsburg, VA: Applied Rehabilitation Concepts.
23. *AssessAbility Users' Guide.* Austin, TX: MediSys Rehabilitation Inc.

24. *The Blankenship System Users' Guide.* Macon, GA: The Blankenship System.
25. *ERGOS Users' Guide.* Tuscon, AZ: Work Recovery Systems Inc.
26. *Isernhagen Work System Users' Guide.* Duluth, MN: Isernhagen Work Systems.
27. *Key Method Users' Guide.* Minneapolis, MN: Key Method.
28. *Physical Work Performance Evaluation Users' Guide.* Birmingham, AL: Ergoscience.
29. *WEST-EPIC Users' Guide.* Ballwin, MO: Employment Potential Improvement Corp.
30. *WorkAbility Mark III Users' Guide.* Ryde, New South Wales, Australia.
31. *WorkHab Users' Guide.* Bundaberg, Queensland, Australia: WorkHab Australia.

part two

Treatment

chapter six

Exercise Rehabilitation for Occupational Low Back Pain

Barbara A. Heller, D.O.

6.1 Overview

Back pain in human beings is extremely common and seemingly a normal part of life. Estimates suggest that 80% of the population will have significant back pain at some time in their lives.[1] Traditional therapy for lower back pain is varied and is usually ineffective. This therapy has included passive modalities (hot packs, electrical stimulation, extended bed rest, and analgesics). These techniques do not cure back pain. They are palliative while the natural healing process runs its course. What is becoming clear, however, is that active exercise is more effective than rest.[2] With injury, inflexibilities and muscle weaknesses may worsen as scar tissue forms, interfering with the ability of the muscle to contract efficiently and move through a normal range of motion. Pain may lessen the intensity and frequency with which the person uses his muscles, causing a downward spiral of further inflexibilities and weakness, possibly leading to recurrent injury. Due to these physical adaptations, efficient biomechanical movements become difficult, leading to a change in movement patterns to avoid pain or because strength, endurance, or flexibility is inadequate to perform the activity or task. This cycle may continue until eventually the worker is unable to successfully complete usual physical tasks or serious injury results.

The intent of this chapter is to describe the components of an active exercise program and examine the possible role of exercise in the treatment of low back pain.

The purpose of exercise in the patient with low back pain and/or leg pain is to enhance healing of the injured structure and to enhance the stability of the spine.

Generally, the concept of spinal instability implies that excessive or inappropriate intervertebral motions cause compression or stretch to inflamed neural elements or injury to ligaments, joint capsules, annular fibers, or end plates of vertebrae, causing pain.[3, 4] Attempts have been made to quantitatively characterize instability as abnormal intervertebral motion (larger or smaller than what is considered to be normal).[5-8] Other hypotheses have suggested that imprecise motion at a joint's axis of rotation may lead to pain.[9, 10] In the shoulder joint, for example, the action of the rotator cuff muscles in maintaining the head of the humerus within its instantaneous axis of rotation within the glenoid is felt to be necessary to ensure proper shoulder function. Loss of precise motion may lead to pain and dysfunction. There have been attempts to relate what has been felt to be abnormal intervertebral motion to low back pain and dysfunction, but the existing studies have arrived at conflicting conclusions.[11, 12]

Panjabi has proposed concepts concerning normal and abnormal function of spinal stabilizers which may be useful in approaching the problem of treating low back pain and/or leg pain.[13]

The spinal stabilizing system is conceptualized by Panjabi as consisting of three subsystems. The first is the passive musculoskeletal system including the vertebrae, facets, discs, and ligaments. The second is the active musculoskeletal system consisting of muscles and tendons. The third is the neural-control system comprised of various tension transducers located in muscle, tendons, and ligaments, as well as more central motor-control centers.

In health, these three subsystems function in an integrated fashion to meet the complex demands applied to the spine. These demands relate to posture, change in load and lever arms, variations in velocity of applied load, and differing loads applied dynamically which are expected versus unexpected.

With injury, degeneration, disease, or disuse, one or more of these subsystems may be adversely affected. The system as a whole, however, appears to have the ability to compensate for the deficits to a degree through adaptive changes and enhancement of existing function.

Panjabi has suggested that a stabilizing compensation of the passive subsystem is the increasing age-related stiffness of the spine due to such structural changes as osteophytic development. These changes are suggested to possibly be in response to reduced muscular strength associated with age and disuse or a dysfunction or deterioration of the active musculoskeletal subsystem.

Successful application of motor-learning principles to train muscles to provide specific directional stability to unstable injured knees through shortening of muscle response time has been demonstrated in the knee literature.[14] This seems to indicate that the neural-control system does have the reserve ability to enhance its function and partially compensate for injury to passive ligamentous structures.

The active musculoskeletal subsystem has a very significant role in stabilizing the spine and protecting the underlying passive elements. If one loads an intact spine complete with ligaments, T1 to the sacrum, a load of only 20 N (2 Kg) is required to buckle the spine or render it unstable.[15] In life, the load-carrying capacity of the human spine is obviously much greater. The added stabilizing forces come largely from the well-coordinated muscles surrounding the spinal column.

Cady et al. demonstrated prospectively that increased strength secondary to training decreased the risk for development of low back pain.[16] Kong et al. recently demonstrated, using a combination of mathematical models, that muscle dysfunction (weakness) did, in fact, reduce the stability of the spinal system, shift loads to the intervertebral discs and ligaments, and decrease the role of the facet joint in transmitting load and stabilizing the spine.[17] Kong suggested that the increased loads applied to the underlying passive structures may lead to potential injury and structural changes to these elements. This study did not answer, however, the question of whether specific strengthening of the muscular system would, in fact, compensate for injury.

The concept of muscular stabilization has been applied successfully in cases of ACL-deficient knees. Giove et al. demonstrated that an increased ratio of hamstring-to-quadriceps strength was the best indication of successful rehabilitation of ACL-deficient knees.[18] This information suggests that strengthening of specific muscle groups may compensate for specific passive instability due to injury.

6.2 Functional Enhancement of the Active Musculoskeletal Subsystem

There exists a growing consensus in the spine literature that exercise is necessary and important for successful rehabilitation of low back injuries.[2] The components of the active subsystem (muscles, tendons) which can be enhanced through active rehabilitation include strength, endurance, range of motion, nutrition, and knowledge of and use of optimal static and dynamic posture. The healing of injured passive and active elements (ligaments, muscles, discs) also can be facilitated through active exercise.

6.2.1 Strength Training

Strength training requires progressive overload of the muscles utilizing fairly high resistance, low repetition, and low duration exercise.[19] Benefits to be gained from strength training from a physiological point of view include improved neuromotor communication, increased musculoskeletal integrity, strength of connective tissue, strength of underlying bone to which the tendons are attached, increased blood flow, and increased tolerance to anaerobic fatigue.[20] The major advantage as demonstrated by Cady is the increased ability of the body to withstand greater applied forces and therefore reduce the risk for injury.[16]

During approximately the first 4 to 6 weeks of training, strength does increase with no actual hypertrophy of muscle fibers. The initial training period resulting in measurable strength gains has been shown to be secondary to adaptations in the maximum neural activation or more efficient nerve-to-muscle communication.[19, 20]

Actual muscle fiber hypertrophy begins around the 6 to 8 week mark of training and continues from that point forward.[19] The importance of continuing a progressive-resistive program beyond two to three weeks of physical therapy becomes obvious.

Suggestions as to why increased muscular strength might prevent injury have been explored. Garrett (1987) demonstrated that maximally stimulated muscle absorbs significantly more energy prior to failure than submaximally or nonstimulated muscle.[21] This may indicate that a stronger muscle may absorb more energy than a weak muscle before reaching the point of muscle strain. Tendons and ligaments demonstrated increased thickness, weight, and strength in response to physical activity. Ligaments have also been shown to heal faster and collagen fibers align properly in response to specific exercise or load.[22–24]

6.2.2   Endurance Training

Aerobic training is typically low resistance, high repetition, and of long duration. Walking or jogging is a good example of aerobic training because it is typically done over a fairly long period of time with little resistance and great repetition. The purpose of endurance training is to develop a more efficient vascular system. The benefits include increased blood flow, decreased peripheral resistance, decreased blood pressure, increased capillarization, increased mitochondrial density, and increased aerobic enzymes in the metabolic chain. The general benefits include better weight management and a better sense of psychological well-being. Of great importance, however, is that endurance training encourages a greater availability of blood flow and oxygen for nutrition and waste removal.[25]

Aerobic conditioning in low-back-injured workers aids the mechanisms of injury repair at the cellular level. In order for optimal tissue repair to occur, good blood flow must reach the injured tissue. It is here that the real action of injury repair occurs. Metabolites of injury must be removed while, at the same time, sufficient oxygen and nutrients are made available. Typically, physical therapy has used passive modalities (i.e., hot packs, ultrasound, etc.) to stimulate blood flow. While the concept of external stimulation seems reasonable (i.e., warming the injured tissue to increase blood flow), the literature suggests that it is of little value. It makes considerably more sense to drive the vascular pump and increase flow from the heart to the injured tissue rather than to try to stimulate it externally. Increased blood flow requires an increase in large-muscle activity via such activities as walking, jogging, bicycling, and swimming.[25]

6.2.3 Range of Motion

It is well-known that early controlled movement of an injured limb reduces adhesions and subsequent contracture development, prevents disuse atrophy, and encourages proper postinjury alignment of connective tissue.[22–24] Inflammation can be minimized by progressive movement of the injured tissue. Early motion leads to the movement of extracellular and extravascular fluid out of the tissue as well as movement of nutritional metabolites into the tissue.

Motion is especially important in regard to nutritional needs of the disc. The nucleus pulposus of the disc is the largest avascular tissue in the body surrounded by the collagenous annulus. Because of the avascular nature of the nucleus, disc hydration and nutrition occur only through the vertebral end plates of the adjacent vertebral bodies. Movement of the vertebral motion segments provides the pumping action required for fluid exchange within the disc and therefore is very important for maintenance of a healthy disc. Perhaps controlled motion may be important for healing of an injured disc as well.

Muscle imbalances and flexibility deficits have been associated with increased injuries in athletic populations.[26] Imprecise motion at a joint's axis of rotation leads to disorders of movement. The concept of longevity and efficiency of a biomechanical system requiring maintenance of precise movement of rotating segments is applied to human movement. The theory suggests that dysfunction may eventually lead to structural changes of underlying passive structures. Pain may be a result of these changes.[9]

In the cervical literature, the clinical relevance of biomechanics is that it describes the normal physiology of the neck. Under normal conditions, the typical cervical vertebrae exhibit a fluid motion. In flexion-extension, each vertebra undergoes an arcuate motion that is produced by simultaneous rotation and horizontal gliding. The geometric center of this arcuate motion is known as the instantaneous axis of rotation (IAR).

The location of IARs for each of the cervical vertebrae has been determined in normal volunteers. They occur in tightly clustered zones around mean locations in the vertebral body below the moving vertebra. The further the IAR lies away from the moving vertebra, the more that vertebra exhibits gliding as opposed to rotation.

Neck pain has been shown to be strongly correlated with abnormally located IARs, but the location of the IAR does not necessarily implicate that segment as the source of pain. IARs can be displaced by such factors as muscle spasm secondary to pain elsewhere in the neck. IARs are an index of the quality of the motion of the neck. This location is determined by the sum of all forces acting on a vertebra. If those forces are changed, the location of the

IAR will change. An abnormal location implies an abnormal balance of forces.[35]

In a multijoint system, movement will occur through the path of least resistance. Stiffness or inflexibility of a muscle defined as resistance to passive stretch (secondary to hypertrophy of the muscle) is theorized to contribute to abnormal or excessive movement at a joint, usually in a specific direction other than the direction in which the movement should primarily occur. A relative hypermobility in the compensatory direction will occur with repetitive use. In other words, if a muscle with multiple actions at more than one joint becomes stiff and inflexible, length for a desired motion may be accomplished by simultaneously performing another motion—a substitution pattern.

A more general example of this type of dysfunction is a situation where hip and pelvic muscles are relatively more stiff/inflexible and hypertrophied (stronger) than the muscles surrounding the lumbar spine. If trunk flexion is the desired motion, movement will occur through the path of least resistance. This will theoretically lead to a subtle increased ratio of lumbar motion/hip motion, suggesting that there is now relatively greater and inappropriate motion or repetitive stress across the compensating lumbar motion segments.

As in the polio era where gross patchy muscle weakness or imbalance led to painful hypermobile unstable joints, relief of pain was accomplished by stabilizing the joints via bracing or arthrodesis. Likewise, the site of pain generation in many lumbar pain syndromes may be the site of relative hypermobility or subtle instability, a consequence of muscle imbalance.[9]

Simplistically stated, treatment involves restoration of proper muscle length, restoration of proper muscle recruitment patterns, improvement of postural alignment with static and functional activities, and improvement of strength imbalances to restore spinal stability.

In 1994, the Agency for Health Care Policy Research (AHCPR) established treatment guidelines for acute low back pain.[36] The guidelines were based on a review of the literature but were not well-accepted by spine treating specialists.

As described by Casazza, Young, and Herring in their recent chapter on the role of exercise in the prevention and management of acute low back pain, the literature did not stand up to careful scrutiny, leading to misconceptions about the benefits of exercise. Concerns with the literature cited by the AHCPR relate to poor description of subjects, poor control of the length of time and number of episodes of back pain prior to intervention, poor distinction regarding whether patients underwent surgery, and lack of acknowledgment of the presence or absence of radiculopathy.[37] It is additionally important to recognize that absence of proof due to methodological flaws in the literature is not equivalent to proof of an absence of beneficial effect of exercise in these patients.

Despite the drawbacks of research trials investigating the efficacy of exercise in the treatment of low back pain, there is mounting clinical evidence of true benefit to rehabilitation. Saal and Saal's retrospective cohort study noting that 90% of patients with herniated lumbar discs attained good-to-excellent results with an aggressive lumbar stabilization program and 92% returned to work is such an example.

6.2.4   *The Exercise Program*

The point of any exercise program is to cause adaptive changes at the cellular level. In other words, a program should be designed to ensure that measurable gains occur in strength and endurance. In regard to posture, the analogy of a car out of alignment leading to early progressive deterioration of parts of the car may intuitively be applied to the potential long-term effects of poor posture on the spine. Similarly, proper alignment of vertebral segments fused by instrumentation is felt by many surgeons to slow the probable future degenerative changes of the unfused segments above and below the fusion. Perhaps the goal of adequate strengthening is to allow and promote optimal individual static and dynamic posture or body use, minimizing repetitive stress across the vertebral motion segments. These issues are difficult to define, investigate, and quantify, however.

The two major principles which govern successful accomplishment of strength and endurance gains are: (1) overload and (2) specificity of training. Proper application of these principles is essential for achievement of these goals.

The principle of overload dictates that for adaptive change to occur in muscle, the muscle must be overloaded or loaded beyond its normal day-to-day activity. Smidt et al. analyzed strength tests and resistive exercises commonly used for trunk strengthening.[27] Using a modeling approach, the conventional sit-up, double straight-leg lowering, and prone trunk extension exercises were found to be poor discriminators of trunk muscle strength, lacking the range of resistance necessary to cover the continuum of human trunk-strength capability. Smidt demonstrated that while doing the most difficult version of each exercise with maximum lever arms, holding an additional 15-pound weight was still required in order to overload the muscle sufficiently to create force equivalent to the average volitional muscle strength capability demonstrated by 38 men on a KinCom isokinetic machine. The point is that once a person can easily do a certain number of prescribed repetitions of an exercise, additional resistance must be progressively added or no further strengthening will occur.

Hakkinen reports in a review article evaluating factors which influence trainability of muscle strength during short-term and prolonged training that resistance as high as 80–120% of a one-repetition maximum (the maximum load a person can lift one time) should be utilized to maximize strengthening.[19]

The prescription for strength or endurance training must also take into account three more principles: frequency, intensity, and duration of the exercise program. The prescription of exercise is an art that is based on scientific principles. Training too seldom will yield little or no benefit. Even if the overload stimulus achieved during each training session is sufficient, too much time between training sessions will allow detraining to occur. Braith et al. showed that training the knee extensors (quadriceps) three times per week was superior to training twice per week for up to 18 weeks of training.[28]

Grave and Pollock found for lumbar extensors, training frequencies between once every two weeks to three times a week were equally effective at improving isometric strength over 12 weeks of training.[29] The literature suggests that once a desired strength or level of endurance has been reached, the frequency of exercise can be decreased with minimal loss of gains through detraining as long as the intensity of exercise remains constant.[29, 30]

The second major principle of specificity has to do with the way in which the physiologic adaptation will occur. It is directly related to the first principle of overload. A simple way to describe this principle is to say that whatever is trained will be enhanced. For example, for arm strength to be gained, arm muscle must be specifically overloaded by increasing resistance against which the muscle exerts force. The concept of muscle substitution in the actual performance of the exercise is an important consideration. Meticulous attention to technique must be observed while exercising. If the goal is to strengthen specifically the lower fibers of the trapezius or the posterior fibers of the gluteus medius muscle, isolated exercises of those muscle groups must be achieved. Motion will occur through the path of least resistance. If close attention is not paid to which muscle is being trained, stronger, more often-used muscles may easily substitute for the little-used, weaker muscle. If substitution occurs, one's goal of specific muscle-group training will have failed.

For endurance to be gained, large muscle overloading aerobic activity must take place. In other words, specific training causes very specific changes to occur. A person will not get stronger doing aerobic training, nor will he gain endurance by strength training. The principle of specificity goes even further to say that one exercise activity does not necessarily transfer well to a different activity. Swimming, for example, does not transfer well to running. If the test used to determine the aerobic capacity of a patient does not reflect the method of training, the test itself may be misleading. Both swimming and jogging may increase the capacity of the cardiovascular system; however, the activities are specific enough that they do not transfer well for testing purposes.

6.2.5 Designing a Rehabilitation Program

Before we can prescribe an effective treatment program, we must have a specific diagnosis. Andersson and McNeill wrote: "It is commonly stated that less than 10% of back pains ever have a diagnosis other than a description of the presenting syndrome. We believe that it is reasonable and proper to relate a given syndrome to the most probable underlying pathology, even though scientific proof does not always exist. This is the only way in which a physician can render reasonable treatment."[31] The American Physical Therapy Association House of Delegates mandated in 1994 that physical therapists also must establish a diagnosis of the condition they are treating. A diagnosis by a therapist is considered to be a syndrome defined by a cluster of signs and symptoms of impairments. The diagnoses must meet scientific standards of reliability and validity.[9]

6.2.6 Consideration of Diagnostic Subsets

1. Discogenic Subsets

   - annular tear
   - HNP
     —without nerve root irritation
     —with nerve root irritation and no neural deficit
     —with nerve root irritation and neural deficit
   - degenerative disc disease
   - internal disc disruption

2. Posterior Element Subsets

   - facet pain syndrome
   - spondylolysis
     —without spondylolisthesis, with and without nerve root irritation
   - spondylolisthesis
     —without nerve root irritation
     —with nerve root irritation and no neural deficit
     —with nerve root irritation and neural deficit
   - stenosis subsets
     —central
     —lateral recess
     —foraminal

3. Segmental Instability
   - with nerve root irritation
   - without nerve root irritation

6.3 The Treatment Program

6.3.1 The Pain-Control Phase

The initial early treatment of acute low back pain involves such interventions as teaching the patient to assume positions of comfort, teaching spine-safe negotiation of position changes such as rising to standing from a chair or getting out of bed, and allowing time-limited relative rest (Figures 6.1–6.3).

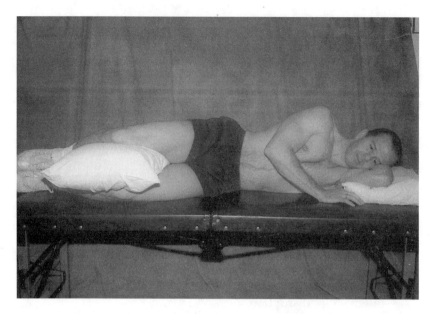

Figure 6.1   Lateral position of lumbar spine rest and comfort.

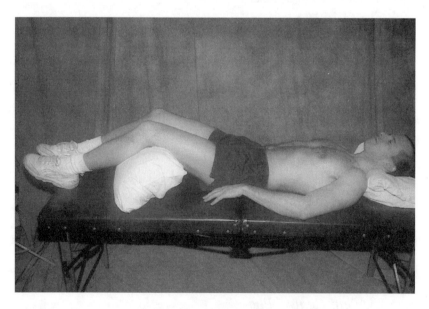

Figure 6.2   Supine position of lumbar spine rest and comfort.

These interventions teach the patient to take some control over his pain. Short-term use of oral medications, passive modalities, and injections may be helpful. Directionally related exercise such as extension exercises can be quite valuable in reducing or centralizing pain in discogenic injury subsets (Figure

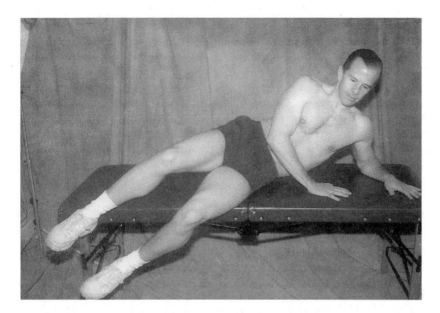

Figure 6.3 Spine-safe position change from supine to side lying to short sitting.

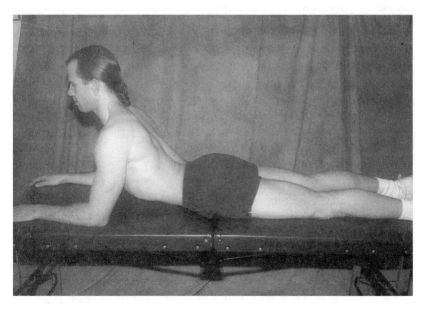

Figure 6.4 Extension exercise to centralize pain in discogenic subsets.

6.4). If extension exercises cause increased extremity pain, however, they are contraindicated. The increased leg pain may indicate the presence of significant bony stenosis or disc herniation in the lateral recess or foraminal or extraforaminal zones.

Flexion-directed exercises initially may be quite helpful with posterior element and stenotic diagnostic subsets. With time, strengthening of muscle groups on both sides of the body becomes important as symptoms dictate.

6.3.2   Training Phase

The training phase promotes enhancement of the musculotendinous and neural-control subsystems to develop adequate strength and endurance in the muscles supporting and protecting the spine.

6.3.3   Diagnosis-Related Decision-Making and the Exercise Prescription

Many, if not most, workers with the acute onset of low back pain and/or leg pain do quite well with time, following the natural history for resolution of their symptoms.

If a patient falls off the natural history course for resolution per episode, a closer look at the treatment program is required. Some researchers, in fact, question whether closely managed appropriate exercise-based rehabilitation might actually change the natural history of low back pain and/or leg pain by decreasing the frequency of recurrences, shortening the duration of discomfort, and decreasing the intensity of episodes.

If a 45-year-old materials handler with low back pain sustained on the job 6 weeks prior fails to report any improvement after physical therapy 3 times a week for 6 weeks, how might one evaluate where the treatment program may have gone wrong? Initially, if one assumes that a specific and correct diagnosis was made attributing the pain to the most likely pain generator and a proper physical therapy prescription was written following exercise physiology principles, then the following questions can be asked:

1. *During the physical therapy program, was there failure to move from the acute pain-control phase to the training phase?* Excessive passive treatments (i.e., heat, ice, manipulation, massage, injections, etc.) may foster the development of a "sick role" in the patient. The worker may adopt an attitude whereby he expects the health care provider to passively "cure" him. This process may lead to the creation of iatrogenic disability. We must remember whose problem it is and function to guide and assist the worker in taking personal responsibility in an active participatory program to improve his function and pain. Just as health problems such as hypertension and diabetes cannot be cured but, instead, become controlled, a similar expectation for control versus lifetime cure of low back pain must be taught to and understood by the patient.
2. *The correct diagnosis was made, the correct exercise program was prescribed, but the execution of the exercises was inappropriate.* Probably one of the most often-cited reasons by patients for stopping their exercise pro-

grams is that the exercises caused more pain. One might regard the patient, therapist, and physician as members of a team with a common goal. In regard to individual exercises, each member should understand the purpose of the exercise and, very importantly, the proper technique for executing exercise. In almost all cases, a particular strengthening goal can be accomplished without undue exacerbation of pain with some alteration in how the exercise is done, if needed. Often the patient simply did not completely understand what the proper exercise technique was and needs to be retaught. Exercises do require a degree of motor learning. Motor learning theory dictates that initially a new motor pattern must be done slowly, broken down into its component parts. Cognitive awareness or thinking about what one is doing must occur before the movement pattern can be done quickly *and correctly.*

A well-meaning lower extremity stretching program may be done inappropriately, directing stretching to the wrong structures. Again, motion will occur through the path of least resistance, and specificity of effort is critical to achieve the desired outcome. Hamstring stretching may be considered as an example. If one sits on the end of the table with one knee extended and a slouched posture with reversal of the lumbar lordotic curve, the goal may be stretching of the hamstrings; but significant range of motion will actually come from the low back as the lordosis reverses (versus stretching the hamstrings). Specific stretching of the hamstring muscles, avoiding substitution by the back muscles, requires maintenance of the lumbar lordosis which is facilitated by simultaneous contraction of the abdominal muscles to truly stabilize the lumbar spine. Stretch then can occur over the two joints that the hamstrings cross—the hip and knee only.

3. *Right diagnosis/wrong exercise program.* If a diagnosis of symptomatic central or lateral (stenosis) or symptomatic spondylolysis is made, extension exercises are contraindicated. Rotation exercises also may be inappropriate as well, secondary to coupled motion.

One should carefully differentiate between a radiological diagnosis of stenosis versus truly symptomatic spinal stenosis. Clinicians who have had experience with over 25,000 patients with low back pain, including some with a radiological diagnosis of stenosis, indicate that they have found lumbar extension strengthening exercises to be very helpful in most patients, achieving treatment goals of increased trunk strength, improved function, and decreased pain.[32]

Symptomatic lateral stenosis, on the other hand, is defined by an increase in leg symptoms in a radicular pattern with progressive walking, relieved by sitting, or partially relieved by walking in a forward-flexed position as when pushing a grocery cart. Symptomatic central stenosis similarly causes increased back pain and possibly buttock pain with walking and is relieved by sitting or walking in a progressively forward-flexed posture, mechanically allowing more room for the thecal sac exiting nerve roots and their respective blood supply. It is with the symptomatic stenotic versus the radiologically defined stenotic patient that extension exercises would generally be contraindicated. In regard to the patient with a new symptomatic spondylolysis, after healing has occurred or extension-related symptoms have resolved, back extensor muscle strengthening should commence.

4. *Right diagnosis/exercise program not advancing as the patient advances.* The only way to strengthen a muscle is by progressively overloading it with resistance. This concept is dictated by the major exercise physiology principle of progressive overload. If a 30-year-old heavy materials handler is asked to do three sets of 10 partial sit-ups, arms across his chest or behind his head, the last repetitions become as easy as the first repetition, and the exercise is not intensified (the resistance the abdominal muscles are called to work against is not progressively increased), no additional strengthening will occur. The principle of progressive overload must be followed with each muscle group strengthened (Figures 6.5–6.10).

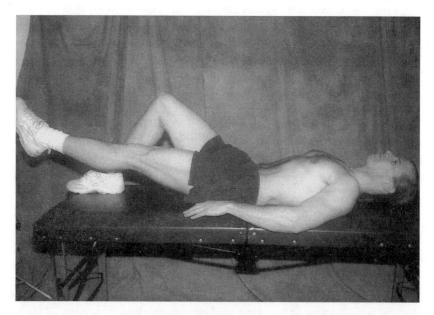

Figures 6.5, 6.6, 6.7, 6.8   Progression of abdominal strengthening following the overload principle, specifically initially increasing the length of the lever arm to increase resistance, then adding external weight to further increase difficulty of exercise.

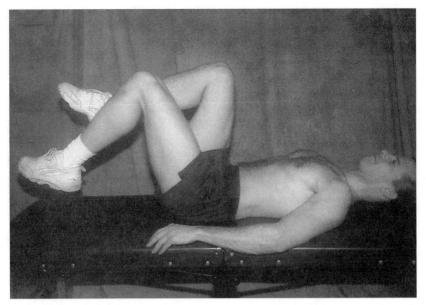

Figure 6.6

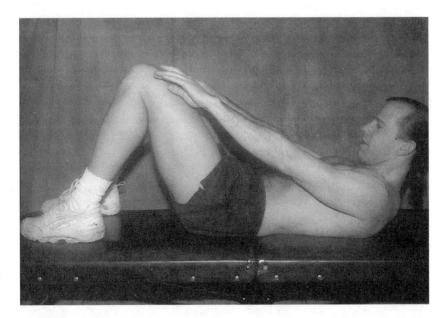

Figure 6.7

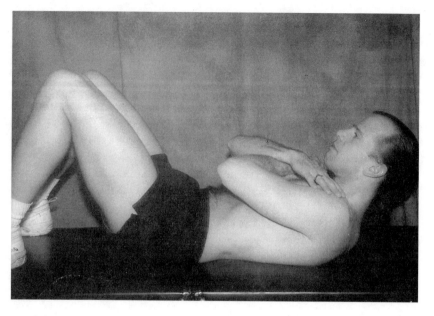

Figure 6.8

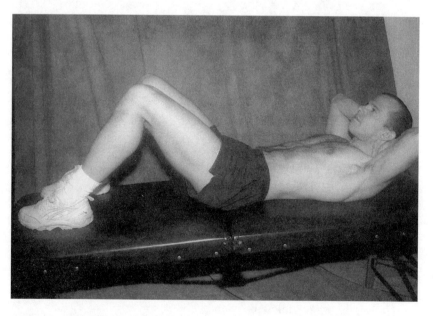

Figures 6.9, 6.10 Progression of lower abdominal strengthening exercise while maintaining a stable lower spine.

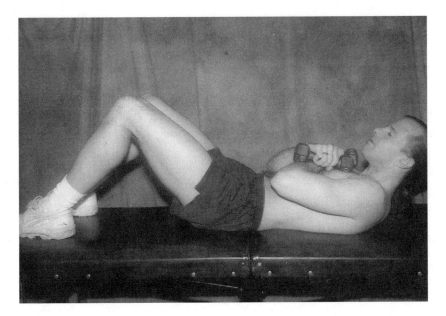

Figure 6.10

5. *Incomplete program.* As stated earlier, the exercise parameters followed to achieve strengthening are different from those used to achieve an increase in endurance. Running or walking on a treadmill, if done in a progressive manner, will increase endurance; but this form of exercise will not strengthen the trunk muscles. Both forms of exercise are important but with differing goals. One must be clear in what one is attempting to achieve with each portion of the exercise program and prescribe the appropriate type of exercise (strength versus endurance), given the goals (Figures 6.11–6.13).

6. *Wrong diagnosis.* If a diagnosis was made attributing the pain to what was felt to be the most likely pain generator, all of the above issues were properly investigated, but the patient is still no better, one must always question whether the correct diagnosis was made initially.

7. *Risk factors for chronic disability.* One must be aware that there may exist nonphysiologic external factors impacting negatively on a patient's ability to improve with both function and pain complaints. A few of the factors to consider are: the presence of a job to return to; litigation pending and other secondary gain issues; a history of physical, psychological, or sexual abuse; a bad evaluation by the patient's supervisor; and the perception on the patient's part that his job is too heavy or difficult.[33]

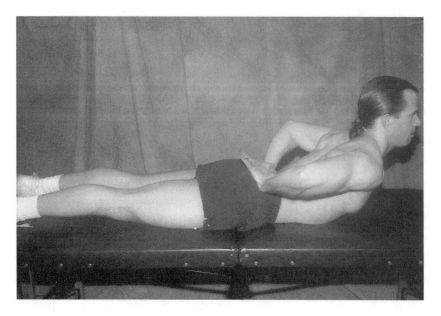

Figure 6.11   Back extensor strengthening.

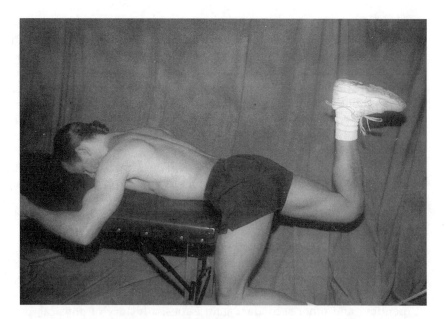

Figure 6.12   Hip abductor strengthening. Note that abdominals are pretightened to prevent movement through the lumbar spine and isolate strengthening to the hip abductors.

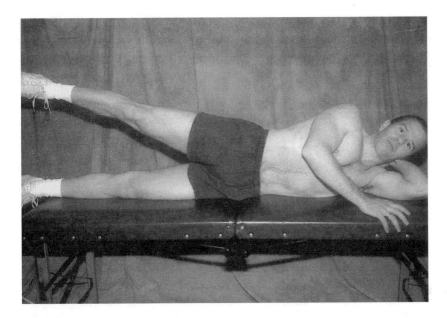

Figure 6.13   Isolated strengthening to hip extensor muscles.

Certain final practical comments in regard to exercise prescription may be helpful. Participating in physical therapy routinely three times a week for a certain number of weeks may not be necessary. As the patient learns to do the exercises well, the visits with the therapist can be spread out to two times a week, to once a week, or perhaps once every other week. The correct frequency of exercise should be followed to avoid detraining, but the patient does not necessarily have to be under the direct supervision of a therapist to do the exercises with proper frequency to avoid detraining. The purpose of the visits is to check that the exercises are being done correctly and to advance the patient as he gains in strength and endurance following the overload and specificity of training principles. When a patient can do the prescribed number of repetitions with ease, then the intensity or amount of resistance must be increased. With added weight, the patient may need to initially decrease repetitions but then slowly work back up to the desired number of repetitions. Intermittent positive reinforcement by the physical therapist can be a very positive force in maintaining patient motivation.

One must also consider the pretraining status of the patient. The weaker the patient is to begin with, the easier it is to strengthen him. The first few weeks of exercise will improve the nerve-muscle activation only. Actual muscle hypertrophy will not occur until six to eight weeks into the strengthening program.[19] If a patient begins with a fairly high base level of strength, additional strengthening will be more difficult; meticulous attention to overloading the muscle in a progressive fashion must be done.

Finally, "The expertise of the staff in treatment delivery is the most important factor in achieving satisfactory results, and lack of expertise leads to an adverse conclusion" (Mitchell et al., *Spine*, 1994).[34]

6.4   References

1. Frymoyer, J. W. Back pain and sciatica, *N. Eng. J. of Med.*, 5:318, 291, 1988.
2. *Clinical Guidelines for Low Back Pain*. Washington, DC: Agency for Health Care Policy and Research, 1994.
3. Wyke, B. The neurological basis of thoracic spine pain, *Rheumatolog. Phys. Med.*, 10:356, 1970.
4. Nachemson, A. Lumbar spine instability: A critical update and symposium summary, *Spine*, 10:290, 1985.
5. Kirkaldy-Willis, W. H. *Managing Low Back Pain*. New York: Churchill Livingstone, 1983.
6. Gertzbein, S. D., Wolfson, N., King, G. The diagnosis of segmental instability in vivo by centrode length. Proceedings of The International Society for The Study of The Lumbar Spine, Miami, 1988.
7. Lehman, T., Brand, R. Instability of the lower lumbar spine. Proceedings of The International Society for The Study of the Lumbar Spine, Toronto, Canada, 1982.
8. Seligman, J., Gertzbein, S., Tile, M. et al. 1984 Volvo award in basic science. Computer analysis of spinal segment motion in degenerative disc disease with and without axial loading, *Spine*, 9:566, 1984.
9. Sahrman, S. Course: Diagnosis and Treatment of Muscle Imbalances Associated with Musculoskeletal Pain Syndromes, Level I and Level III, School of Physical Therapy, Washington University, St. Louis, MO, January, 1997.
10. Kibler, W. B., Chandler, T. J. Role of scapula in the overhead throwing motion, *Contemporary Orthoped.*, vol 22. 6:525, 1991.
11. Pearcy, M., Shepherd, J. Is there instability in spondylolisthesis? *Spine*, 10:175, 1985.
12. Dvorak, J., Panjabi, M. M., Novotny, J. E. et al. Clinical validation of functional flexion-extension roentgenograms of the lumbar spine, *Spine*, 16:943, 1991.
13. Panjabi, M. M. The stabilizing system of the spine, Part 1: Function, dysfunction, adaptation, and enhancement, *J. of Spinal Disorders*, 5:383, 1992.
14. Ihara, H., Nakayama, A. Dynamic joint control training for knee ligament injuries, *Amer. J. of Sports Med.*, 14:309, 1986.
15. Lucas, D. B., Bresler, B. Stability of the ligamentous spine. Technical Report esr 11, no. 40, Biomechanics Laboratory, University of California at San Francisco, The Laboratory.
16. Cady, L. D., Bischoff, D.P., O'Connel, E. R. et al. Strength, fitness and subsequent back injuries in firefighters, *J. of Occup. Med.* 21: 269, 1979.
17. Kong, W. Z., Goel, V. K., Gilbertson, L. G. et al. Effects of muscle dysfunction on lumbar spine mechanics. A finite element study based on a two-motion segment mode, *Spine*, 1:19, 2197, 1996.
18. Giove, T. P., Miller, S. J., Kent, B. E. et al. Nonoperative treatment of the torn anterior cruciate ligament, *J. of Bone and J. Surg.*, 65A, 184, 1983.
19. Hakkinen, K. Factors influencing trainability of muscular strength during short-term and prolonged training, *Nat. Strength and Cond. Assoc. J.*, 7:2, 32, 1985.

20. Horitani, T., DeVries, H. A. Neural factors versus hypertrophy in the time course of muscle strength gains, *Amer. J. of Phys. Med.*, 58:3, 115, 1979.
21. Garrett, W. E., Safran, M. R., Seaber, A. V. et al. Biomechanical comparison of stimulated and nonstimulated skeletal muscle pulled to failure, *Amer. J. of Sports Med.*, 15(5), 448, 1987.
22. Staff, P. H. The effect of physical activity on joints, cartilage, tendons, and ligaments, *Scand. J. of Soc. Med.*, 29 (suppl), 59, 1982.
23. Tipton, C. M., James, S. L., Mergner, W. et al. Influence of exercise on strength of medial collateral knee ligaments of dogs. *Amer. J. of Phys.*, 218 (3), 894, 1970.
24. Tipton, C. M., Matthes, R. D., Maynard, J. A. et al. The influence of physical activity on ligaments and tendons, *Med. and Sci. in Sports*, 7:165, 1975.
25. Sharkey, B. J. Intensity and duration of training and the development of cardiorespiratory endurance, *Med. Sci. and Sports*, 2, 1970.
26. Chandler, T. J., Kibler, W. B., Wooten, B. et al. Flexibility comparisons of junior elite tennis players to other athletes, *Amer. J. of Sports Med.*, 18 (2), 134, 1990.
27. Smidt, G. L., Blanpied, P. R. Analysis of strength tests and resistive exercises commonly used for low-back disorders, *Spine*, 12:10, 1025, 1987.
28. Braith, R. W., Graves, J. E., Pollock, M. L. et al. Comparison of two vs. three days/weeks of variable resistance training during 10- and 18-week programs, International Journal of *Sports Med.*, 10:450, 1989.
29. Graves, J. E., Pollock, M. L., Foster, D. et al. Effect of training frequency and specificity on isometric lumbar extension strength, *Spine*, 15, 6, 504, 1990.
30. Graves, J. E., Pollock, M. L., Leggett, S. H. et al. Effect of reduced training frequency on muscular strength, *Int. J. of Sports Med.*, 9:316, 1988.
31. Andersson, G. B., McNeill, T. W. *Lumbar Spine Syndromes*, Springer-Verlag: 1989.
32. Personal Communication, Dr. Ted Dreissinger, regarding multicenter experience, Columbia Spine Center.
33. Snook, S. The costs of back pain in industry, *Spine: State of the Art Rev.*, vol. 2, 1, 1, 1987.
34. Mitchel, R. I., Carmen, G. M. The functional restoration approach to the treatment of chronic pain in patients with soft tissue and back injuries, *Spine*, vol. 19, 6, 633, 1994.
35. Bogduk, N. Combined Meeting of the International Spinal Injection Society and the Australasian Faculty of Musculoskeletal Medicine, 1998 Annual Scientific Meeting, Sydney, Australia.
36. Agency for Health Care Policy and Research. *Clinical Practice Guidelines for Acute Low Back Pain*. Rockville, MD: AHCPR, 1994.
37. Casazza, B. A., Young, I. L., Herring, S. A. The Role of Exercise in the Prevention and Management of Acute Low Back Pain. *Occup. Med.: State of the Art Rev.*, vol. 13, #1, January-March, 1998.

chapter seven

The Use of Medications in the Treatment of Low Back Pain

Gerard A. Malanga, M.D.

7.1 Overview

Medications are commonly used in the treatment of low back pain, and can be quite helpful when properly prescribed. Pain is generally the chief complaint of individuals experiencing low back problems and therefore, successful control of pain is an essential initial goal in treatment. Pain; however, should be regarded as a component of a *symptom complex* resulting from an underlying pathological process affecting the low back.[1] The clinician caring for the back pain patient should also strive to establish a *diagnosis* which includes an identification of the causative disorder using an understanding of functional anatomy, biomechanics, and kinesiology in localizing the patient's pain generator(s). At the tissue level this may include bone, disc, tendon, muscle, ligament, or nerve. The process may be biomechanical, inflammatory, infectious, neoplastic, or perhaps psychological in nature (or a combination of factors). By properly determining the tissue(s) involved and the most likely process causing the patient's pain, then the physician can be guided toward the proper initial treatment of the patient, including the most appropriate choice of medications prescribed. By applying the principles of medication use in other musculoskeletal disorders, we can strategically plan the appropriate use of pharmacological agents.

In this chapter, several classes of commonly prescribed drugs for the treatment of low back pain will be reviewed. The mechanisms of action, efficacy and current clinical research, dosing and cost, complications, and contraindications of each will be presented.

7.2   Acetaminophen

Acetaminophen is the principle member of the group of drugs classified as para-aminophenol derivatives. In 1949, acetaminophen became recognized as the primary active metabolite of both acetanilide and phenacetin and has now become a popular and clinically proven analgesic and antipyretic.[2]

While acetaminophen's analgesic and antipyretic effects are equal to those of aspirin, its anti-inflammatory effects are weak. Its therapeutic effects appear to be secondary to an inhibition of prostaglandin biosynthesis with a resultant increase in the pain threshold and modulation of the hypothalamic heat regulating center. The effects of acetaminophen are noted predominantly centrally and less peripherally, where it serves as only a weak inhibitor of cyclooxygenase and does not inhibit the activation of neutrophils as do other NSAIDs.[3]

In the setting of acute low back pain, acetaminophen can be effectively utilized as an analgesic. Several studies have shown acetaminophen to be superior to placebos in the treatment of osteoarthritis pain and it has been recommended as a first-line agent in osteoarthritis treatment.[4, 5, 6] Bradley et al. compared the analgesic properties of acetaminophen to ibuprofen in the treatment of pain associated with osteoarthritis of the knee. Acetaminophen was found to be as efficacious as both low-dose analgesic and high dose anti-inflammatory regimens of ibuprofen in providing pain relief and improving functional outcome during the four-week study period.[7] In a 1982 study, paracetamol, a compound similar to acetaminophen, was compared to diflunisal and a salicylate derivative, in the treatment of chronic low back pain. Thirty patients with a six-month to several-year history of low back pain presumed secondary to facet pathology were treated in a randomized fashion for 4 weeks, and more favorable outcomes were associated with NSAID use.[8]

The accepted oral dose of acetaminophen is 325 to 1,000 mg every 4 to 6 hours, with a 24-hour maximal dose of 4,000 mg. Peak plasma levels and analgesic effects are typically noted from 30 to 60 minutes following ingestion. Acetaminophen is generally available without prescription and is relatively inexpensive.[4] While erythematous or urticarial skin rashes are occasionally observed, the most serious adverse affect of acute acetaminophen overdose is hepatotoxicity. In adults, hepatotoxicity may result from a single dose of 10 to 15 grams. More chronic abuse of acetaminophen has been associated with nephrotoxicity.[2, 3]

Acetaminophen's analgesic effects make it an acceptable medication in the treatment of acute low back pain. It is inexpensive and its use is typically without complications. While effective against mild to moderate pain in some acute back pain situations, it does not offer the patient other desirable effects against inflammation, muscle spasm, or sleep disturbance. It is unlikely to be effective in low back disorders associated with severe pain.

7.3 NSAIDs

Aspirin is the prototypical member of the group of medications known as nonsteroidal anti-inflammatory drugs (NSAIDs). Products of salicin, first isolated from willow bark in 1829, were converted to acetylsalicylic acid, which became recognized for its anti-inflammatory effects and was introduced as aspirin in 1899.[4] In 1984, nearly one in seven Americans were treated with an anti-inflammatory agent, and in 1986, nearly 100 million prescriptions for NSAIDs were written, resulting in worldwide annual sales estimated at $1 billion.[9, 10]

The primary mechanism of action NSAIDs is a reduction of cyclooxygenase activity and a resultant decrease in prostaglandin synthesis. Prostaglandins are active mediators of the inflammatory cascade which also serve to sensitize peripheral nociceptors. A reduction in their local concentration could therefore explain the combined anti-inflammatory and analgesic properties of NSAIDs[11] In single doses, most of the NSAIDs are more effective analgesics than a single dose of acetaminophen or aspirin.[12] Locally, NSAIDs are also felt to combat inflammation by inhibiting neutrophil function and interfering with the activity of enzymes such as phospholipase C.[9] Most NSAIDs do not decrease the production of lipoxygenase-produced leukotrienes, which are also believed to significantly contribute to the inflammatory response.[4] A disparity between the anti-inflammatory and analgesic potencies of these agents in clinical practice has been observed, and recent data has suggested that pain relief from NSAIDs may in part be secondary to a more central antinociceptive component.[13, 14, 15, 16] Measurable levels of anti-inflammatory agents have been detected in the CSF following short-term administration in the setting of a soft-tissue injury.[17]

Aspirin inhibits cyclooxygenase irreversibly through acetylation, whereas several groups of organic acids, including proprionic acid derivatives, acetic acid derivatives, and enolic acids, all of which bind to and reversibly inhibit cyclooxygenase[4] (Table 7.1). Elimination half-lives of these drugs range from less than four hours for some proprionic acid derivatives to greater than 40 hours for piroxicam.[11]

In a recent survey by McCormack and Brune of 26 studies investigating the role of NSAIDs in acute soft-tissue injuries, 14 double-blind placebo-controlled studies were found to demonstrate a significant difference between NSAIDs and placebos for nine NSAIDs — clonixin, ketoprofen, naproxen, diclofenac, fenbufen, ibuprofen, indomethacin, piroxicam, and azapropazone. In those studies where physical therapy was also administered, four NSAIDs — azapropazone, clonixin, naproxen, and ketoprofen — were demonstrated to provide unequivocal additional benefit.[18] In a similar review of investigations of NSAIDs and sports-related soft tissue injuries, Weiler concluded that benefits were typically observed amongst treatment groups when compared with controls. These short-term studies have found that treated athletes return to practice quicker and without any apparent

Table 7.1

Drug and Family	Max Daily Dose (mg)	Usual Single Dose (mg)	Dosing	Half-Life (Hours)	$/Month
Salicylates					
Aspirin	4,000	500–1000	q4–6h	12	15
Nonacetylated Salicylates					
Salsalate (Disalcid, others)	4,000	1,000	q8–12h	16	30
Diflunisal (Dolobid)	1,500	1,000, 500	q8–12h	8–12	30–45
Choline Mg trisalicylate (Trilisate)	3,000	1,000–1,500	q8–12h	9–17	40–120
Proprionic Acids					
Ibuprofen (Motrin, others)	2,400	200–400	q4–6h	2	30–80
Flurbiprofen (Ansaid)	300	50–100	q6–8h	5.7	50–150
Fenoprofen (Nalfon)	1,200	200	q4–6h	3	50–125
Ketoprofen (Orudis, others)	300	25–75	q4–8h	2–4	90–180
Naproxen (Naprosyn)	1,250	500, 250	q6–8h	13	44–80
Naproxen Na (Anaprox)	1,375	550, 275	q12h	13	44–80
Indoles					
Indomethacin (Indocin)	150	25–50	q6–8h	4.5	35–100
Sulindac (Clinoril)	400	150–200	q12h	8	45–90
Tolmetin (Tolectin)	1,800	150–600	q6–8h	2–5	30–90
Etodolac (Lodine)	1,200	200–400	q6–8h	3–11	70–175
Fenamates					
Meclofenamate (Meclomen)	400	100	q6–8h	2	54–162
Others					
Piroxicam (Feldene)	40	20	q24h	50	80–160
Nabumetone (Relafen)	2,000	1,000	q12–24h	24	60–120
Ketorolac (Toradol)	40	10	q6h	4–7	60–120
Oxaprozin (Daypro)	1,800	1,200	q24h	24	70–120

(1, 3, 11, 12, 63)

significant delay in the injury healing process.[10] In 1987, Amlie et al. studied the effects of seven days of oral piroxicam treatment in 278 patients with acute low back pain. Medication administration was commenced within 48 hours of symptom onset, and after three days of therapy, patients in the treatment group revealed a significant amount of pain relief. After seven days, the difference in pain symptoms between the treatment and control groups were no longer significant, but the treatment group demonstrated a significantly lower requirement for additional analgesics and a greater return to work rate.[19] In a 1981 study, patients with rheumatoid arthritis were found to experience little difference in symptom relief when treated with six individual NSAIDs, while in patients with ankylosing spondylitis, naproxen, indomethacin, and fenoprofen were found to be most effective.[20]

The dosing and cost of each NSAID varies significantly by chemical family and agent (Table 7.1). The choice of initial anti-inflammatory agent remains largely empirical. Aspirin is generally very inexpensive, while the newer NSAIDs often cost significantly more. In addition to cost considerations, patients have been observed to be more compliant with those agents which require less frequent dosing.[20] Since steady states of plasma concentration are not typically observed until dosing has been continued for a period of three to five half-lives, plateau concentrations and maximal therapeutic effects are not realized as quickly in those agents with longer half-lives unless a loading dose is first prescribed.[9] By first prescribing a loading dose (which is not often done in clinical settings) and then maintaining regular dosing as indicated for each agent, adequate plasm levels will be achieved for the anti-inflammatory abilities of these medications to be realized. Prescribing NSAIDs in lower dosages and on a less regular schedule is more likely to utilize only the analgesic properties of these agents.[9, 10] Large variations in patient response to different NSAIDs are observed even when chemically similar drugs of a common family are prescribed.[4] Over a one- to two-week period, the dose may be increased to the recommended maximum, and after that time, if the results remain unsatisfactory, a different agent should be tried.[9] Side effects generally develop within the initial weeks of treatment, although gastric complications can develop at later times. Combination therapy with more than one NSAID is to be avoided as the incidence of side effects is additive and there is little evidence of added benefit to the patient.[4]

Several complications are associated with NSAID use. As nonselective inhibitors of cyclooxygenase-2 (COX-2), whose activity is induced in the setting of active inflammation, and cyclooxygenase-1 (COX-1), which is responsible for thromboxane and prostaglandin synthesis and the maintenance of normal gastrointestinal mucosa, NSAIDs are commonly observed to alter gastrointestinal physiology. While dyspepsia is a very common complication, erosion, ulceration, and hemorrhage may also develop and without warning symptoms.[2, 9] The development of NSAIDs that selectively inhibit COX-2 would theoretically provide a much safer anti-inflammatory agent. There is some evidence that nabumetone, which preferentially inhibits COX-2, is associated with a lower incidence of gastrointestinal side effects.[21] Misoprostol, a synthetic prostaglandin E1 analog, has been shown to reduce the likelihood of gastroduodenal erosion during the administration of aspirin.[22] As prostaglandins also participate in the autoregulation of renal blood flow and glomerular filtration, numerous renal side effects, including acute renal failure, have been associated with NSAID use. The kidneys are most vulnerable in those individuals who are in a hypovolemic state or in whom there is preexisting renal disease.[9] While the association between NSAID use and minimal change glomerulonephropathy has been recognized, a recent study suggests that nephrotic syndrome due to membranous nephropathy should also be recognized as a possible adverse reaction to NSAID use.[23] All NSAIDs can cause central nervous system side effects such as drowsiness, dizziness, and confusion.[12] Blockade of platelet aggregation, inhibition of uterine contractility, interference with antihypertensive medications, and hypersensitivity reactions are also side effects shared by many of the commonly prescribed anti-inflammatory agents.[4] Some variability, with regard to adverse effects, has been recognized amongst the NSAIDs. While the nonacetylated salicylates do not prolong bleeding time and have rarely been associated with gastrointestinal complications, indomethacin has more frequently been associated with nausea, gastrointestinal bleeding, and headaches.[24] NSAIDs have less potential for abuse than opioids, and physical dependence on nonsteroidals has not been reported.[12]

Recent studies have investigated the effects of NSAID use upon the healing process of injured soft tissues, in particular, muscles and tendons, which they are often prescribed to treat. Almekinders investigated the in vitro effects of indomethacin on isolated human fibroblasts subjected to repetitive motion injury. NSAID use in this study was associated with decreased DNA synthesis during the early proliferative healing phase but with increased protein synthesis during the later remodeling phase of healing.[25] In an earlier investigation of the effects of piroxicam on the healing of rat tibialis anterior muscle subjected to strain injury, histological observation revealed a delay in the early inflammatory reactions and regeneration within the muscle tissue of the treated group. At 11 days following injury, however, both treated and controlled groups demonstrated similar extents of regeneration and failure loads.[26] A study investigating the effects of flurbiprofen treatment on the recovery of eccentrically injured rabbit muscle revealed treated muscles to demonstrate initial histological and contractile gains but a subsequent functional loss.[27] The effect of NSAIDs upon chondrocyte function and the cartilage matrix has similarly been investigated.[24] As these apparently time dependent effects of NSAID use on soft tissue recovery are further realized, a more scientific approach to the prescription of anti-inflammatory agents will likely arise.

Patients are most likely to benefit from their combined analgesic and anti-inflammatory properties of NSAIDs during the first week after injury onset. The anti-inflammatory properties of these agents are most likely to be realized when therapy is initiated with a loading dose and the recommended dosages are then continued at regular intervals. The prescribing physician needs to be aware of the adverse effects often associated with NSAID use. Prolonged use of anti-inflammatory medications, i.e., greater than three to four weeks in the setting of acute low back pain is generally not indicated.

7.4 Muscle Relaxants

In 1946, the discovery of mephenesin created an interest in medications which produced reversible paralysis in animals without gross sedation. With mephenesin as their prototype, muscle relaxants, which are thought to relax skeletal muscle through actions on the central nervous system (CNS) (Table 7.2), have evolved over the past decades.[29] The muscle relaxing properties of these agents do not arise from direct activity at the muscular or neuromuscular junction level but rather from an inhibition of more central polysynaptic neuronal events. These agents have also been shown in some studies to demonstrate superior analgesia to either acetaminophen or aspirin, and it remains uncertain if muscle spasm is a prerequisite to their effectiveness as analgesics.[11] Muscle relaxants are now often prescribed in the treatment of acute low back pain in an attempt to improve the initial limitations in range of motion from muscle spasm and to interrupt the pain-spasm-pain cycle. Limiting muscle spasm and improving range of motion will prepare the patient for therapeutic exercise.[29]

In an attempt to determine the mechanism of action of carisoprodol in the treatment of low back pain, a double-blind study was carried out comparing its effectiveness to that of a sedative control, butabarbital, and a placebo in the treatment of 48 laborers with acute lumbar pain. Carisoprodol

Table 7.2

Medication	Mechanism of Action	Dosage	Contraindications
Muscle Relaxants			
Carisoprodol (Soma)	Blockage of interneuronal activity in reticular formation and spinal cord	350 mg tid and hs	Acute intermittent porphyria
Chlorzoxazone (Parafon Forte)	Inhibition of polysynaptic reflex arcs at subcortical and spinal cord levels	250–750 mg tid-qid	
Cyclobenzaprine (Flexeril)	Inhibition of alpha and gamma motor neuron activity at brainstem level	10 mg tid	Cardiac disease, hyperthyroidism, use with MAO inhibitors
Methocarbamol (Robaxin)	Unknown, possible general central nervous system depression	1,000–1,500 mg qid	
Benzodiazepines			
Diazepam (Valium)	Depresses activity in limbic system, thalamus, hypothalamus	2–10 mg tid-qid	Acute narrow angle glaucoma

(2, 11)

was found to be significantly more effective in providing both subjective pain relief and objective improvements in range of motion when evaluated by finger to floor testing. The results of this study suggest that the effects of carisoprodol are not secondary to its sedative effects alone.[30]

In 1989, Basmajian compared the effectiveness of cyclobenzaprine alone with diflunisal, placebo, and a combination of cylcobenzaprine and diflunisal in the treatment of acute low back pain and spasm. During the 10-day study period, the combined treatment group demonstrated significantly superior improvements in global ratings on Day 4, but not on Day 2 nor 7. This study suggested some effectiveness of combined analgesic and muscle relaxant therapy when utilized early in initial week of pain onset.[31] Borenstein compared the effects of combined cyclobenzaprine and naproxen with naproxen alone and also found combination therapy to be superior in reducing tenderness, spasm and range of motion in patients presenting with 10 days or less of low back pain and spasm. Adverse effects, predominantly drowsiness, were noted in 12 of 20 in the combined group and only four of 20 treated with naproxen alone.[32]

Cyclobenzaprine and carisoprodol were compared in the treatment of patients with acute thoracolumbar pain and spasm rated moderate to severe and of no longer than seven days' duration. Both drugs were found to be effective, without significant differences between the treatment groups. Significant improvements were noted in physician-rated mobility and in patients' visual analogue scores on followup Days 4 and 8. While 60% of patients experienced adverse effects in the form of drowsiness or fatigue, these differences were not significantly different between groups, and only 8% of patients from each group discontinued treatment.[29] Baratta found cyclobenzaprine, 10 mg tid, superior to placebo in a randomized, double-blind study of 120 patients with acute low back pain presenting within five days of symptom onset. Significant improvement was noted in range of motion, tenderness to palpation, and pain scores on follow up Days 2 through 9. Sixty percent of treatment group patients reported associated drowsiness or dizziness compared with 25% of those in the placebo group.[33]

Although benzodiazepenes are felt to be effective muscle relaxants, there is no scientific evidence to support their use in patients with low back pain. Diazepam was found to offer no significant subjective nor objective benefit, when compared to placebo, in patients treated for low back pain.[34] Carisoprodol was found to be superior to diazepam in the treatment of patients with "at least moderately severe" low back pain and spasm of no longer than seven days' duration. In this study, the overall incidence of adverse reactions was higher in the diazepam treated group but was not of statistical significance.[35]

Muscle spasm of local origin needs to be clinically differentiated from spasticity and sustained muscle contraction in the setting of CNS and upper motor neuron injury. Baclofen (Lioresal) and dantrolene sodium (Dantrium) are two agents whose use is indicated in the setting of spasticity of CNS etiology. Dantrolene sodium is of particular interest, as its mechanism of action is purely at the muscular level where it serves to inhibit the release of calcium from the sarcoplasmic reticulum.[4] Casale studied the effectiveness of dantrolene sodium, 25 mg daily, in the treatment of low back pain and found patients to demonstrate significant improvements in visual analogue scores, pain behavior, and EMG evaluations of "antalgic reflex motor unit firing," when compared with the placebo group. The findings of this study are interesting in that they demonstrate improvement secondary to a pure muscle relaxant which does not possess other outside antinociceptive properties.[36] Baclofen is a derivative of gamma-aminobutric acid (GABA) and is believed to inhibit mono- and polysynaptic reflexes at the spinal level.[4] Treatment with baclofen was compared to placebo in a double-blind, randomized study of 200 patients with acute low back pain.[37] Patients with initially severe discomfort were found to benefit from baclofen, 30 to 80 mg daily, on Days 4 and 10 of follow-up. Forty-nine percent of treatment patients complained of sleepiness, 38% of nausea, and 17% discontinued treatment.

Muscle relaxants (Table 7.2) have gained wide acceptance in the treatment of acute musculoskeletal pain with sedation the most commonly reported side effect. These drugs should be used with caution in patients driving motor vehicles or operating heavy machinery. More absolute contraindications do exist to the use of carisoprodol, cyclobenzaprine, and diazepam. Rare idiosyncratic reactions have also been reported to carisoprodol and its metabolites such as meprobamate.[4] Benzodiazepams have potential for abuse and their use should be avoided. By initially prescribing muscle relaxants at bedtime, the physician can take advantage of their sedative effects and minimize daytime drowsiness. These agents have been found to be effective when used either alone or in combination with an analgesic/anti-inflammatory agent within seven days of symptom onset. The prescribing physician should monitor patients receiving these medications and tailor dosages in an attempt to minimize the drowsiness and sedation often associated with their use. The use of benzodiazepines does not appear to offer any significant benefit to patients experiencing acute low back pain. Further research is needed before the role of baclofen and dantrolene sodium in the treatment of muscle spasm of local origin can be more clearly defined.

7.5 Opioids

Opioids occupy the second rung on the World Health Organization analgesic ladder in the treatment of moderate to severe cancer pain and are commonly prescribed for postoperative pain, where they have been found to successfully treat both local and more generalized pain symptoms.[11]

Opioid drugs produce analgesia by binding to multiple types of opioid receptors which are typically bound by endogenous opioid compounds. These receptors are generally classified as mu, kappa, and delta, but the opioid medications typically prescribed are morphine-like agonists which occupy the mu receptor. These receptors are located both peripherally, on sensory nerves and immune cells, and centrally, in the spinal cord and brainstem.[11]

In a study by Brown et al., the analgesic efficacy of diflunisal, 500 mg PO bid following a 1,000 mg loading dose, was compared to that of 300 mg of acetaminophen with 30 mg of codeine in the treatment of pain resulting from initial or recurrent low back strains. Over this 15-day trial, the analgesic efficacy each regimen was found to be similar, but patient acceptability and tolerance were found to be superior for diflunisal. Five of 21 patients treated with acetaminophen and codeine reported adverse effects including drowsiness, dizziness, fatigue, and nausea, compared with three of 19 patients treated with diflunisal.[38] In a study of 200 patients presenting with acute low back strain, Weisel, et al., compared the analgesic efficacy of acetaminophen with both codeine and aspirin plus oxycodone. A significantly greater pain reduction, especially within the first three days of treatment, was noted for those individuals treated with codeine or aspirin plus oxycodone.[39] None of these medications resulted in a more prompt return to work.

Additional studies have compared opioids with other analgesics in the setting of postoperative pain. Cooper found acetaminophen, 1,000 mg, in combination with oxycodone, 10 mg, to provide superior analgesia to the two combined at lower doses or either drug alone in patients experiencing postoperative dental pain.[40] Acetaminophen was found to be a superior analgesic to propoxyphene in a study of 200 postpartum patients status post-episiotomy.[41] It is unclear how the results of these studies can be extrapolated to pain relief in patients with low back pain.

For most opioids, peak drug effect occurs within one and one-half to two hours following oral administration, and a second opioid dose can safely be taken two hours after the first if side effects are mild at that time. Sustained-release tablets are also available and often prove beneficial in those patients with more rapidly fluctuating pain.[64] The potency of the opioid agonists are generally compared with that of morphine (Table 7.3).

The goal of successful opioid prescription involves achieving a tolerable balance between analgesia and the side effects often associated with opioid

Table 7.3

Agonist Drug	Oral Dose (mg) Equianalgesic to 20–30 mg Morphine
Morphine (MSIR/MS Contin)	20–30
Oxycodone (Percocet*)	20
Hydromorphone (Dilaudid)	1.5
Methadone (Dolophine)	10
Meperidine (Demerol)	75
Levorphanol (Levo-Dromoran)	2

*combination tablet contains acetaminophen

use. Tolerance to adverse effects such as somnolence, nausea, and impaired thought processes typically occurs within days to weeks of initial opioid administration. Constipation is a more persistent side effect which can be managed with stool softeners and laxatives. Normeperidine, a metabolite of meperidine, accumulation with repetitive dosing has been associated with the development of anxiety, tremors, myoclonus, and generalized seizures. Patients with impaired renal function are at particular risk.[47] Methadone demonstrates good oral potency and a plasma half-life of 24–36 hours. Accumulation of methadone may occur with repetitive dosing, resulting in excessive sedation on Days 2 to 5.[64] Physical dependence can develop after several days of administration of opioid analgesics.[11]

Despite the stigmas and fears of addiction associated with their use, when properly utilized by a knowledgeable physician, opioid analgesics successfully treat otherwise intractable pain. The potential role of opioids in the treatment of nonmalignant acute low back pain is limited. They should be reserved for those patients who have either failed to realize adequate analgesia from alternative medications, i.e., NSAIDs plus or minus a muscle relaxant, or who have contraindications to the use of other analgesics. If opioids are prescribed, a regular, rather than a PRN, dosing schedule should be prescribed, and their use should be limited to the first several days following pain onset. The prescribing physician should be aware of the possibility of dependence with more prolonged use and avoid prescribing these agents for those patients with a prior history of substance abuse.

Tramadol hydrochloride is a newer centrally acting analgesic which, although not chemically related to opiates, binds to mu receptors. Its mechanism of action is not completely understood, but is felt to be at least in part secondary to its inhibition of the reuptake of both serotonin and norepinephrine. Tramadol has been demonstrated to provide superior analgesia to combined acetaminophen-propoxyphene in patients experiencing severe postoperative pain, and similar analgesia, but with greater tolerability, to morphine in patients hospitalized for cancer pain.[42, 43] In a four-week study of 390 elderly patients with chronic pain secondary to a variety of conditions, tramadol was found to provide comparable analgesia to acetaminophen with codeine without a significant difference in associated adverse effects.[44] Additional studies reveal the low abuse potential and the absence of significant respiratory depression associated with tramadol use.[45, 46] Individualization of tramadol dosage is recommended for those individuals who are either over 75 years of age, who have impaired renal function, or who have significant liver disease.

7.6   Antidepressants

The antidepressants most commonly prescribed in the U.S. include the tricyclic antidepressants (TCAs) and the newer serotonin reuptake inhibitors (SSRIs). Amitriptyline, imipramine, nortriptyline, and desipramine are representative of the TCAs, which mediate their antidepressant effects through a variable presynaptic inhibition of norepinephrine and serotonin reuptake. Fluoxetine, paroxetine, and sertraline are commonly prescribed SSRIs which, as their name indicates, act by specifically blocking the reuptake of serotonin by the presynaptic terminal. Monoamine oxidase inhibitors (MAOIs) inhibit the activity of monoamine oxidase and thereby increase the concentrations of endogenous norepinephrine, serotonin, and epinephrine in the nervous system.[56]

While several classes of antidepressants have been used successfully in the treatment of a variety of pain syndromes, the literature most strongly supports the analgesic efficacy of the tricyclics. Amitriptyline has been investigated as an analgesic more than the other antidepressant agents and appears to be the most popular antidepressant analgesic in the clinical setting. Migraine headaches, neuropathic pain associated with diabetic neuropathy, and postherpetic neuralgia have been found to respond favorably to antidepressant administration. These agents have also been found to alleviate the pain associated with musculoskeletal conditions such as fibromyalgia, rheumatoid arthritis, and osteoarthritis.[57] Antidepressants have been successfully utilized in the treatment of cancer pain. In the cancer population, when administered concurrently with an antidepressant, opioid agents may be used at a reduced dose and with a diminished incidence of side effects.[58]

The analgesic abilities of antidepressants were once felt to be related to the alleviation of the depression which can often accompany persistent pain, but several antidepressants have been found to reduce pain symptoms in patients not experiencing comorbid depression.[57] These agents are now believed to have primary analgesic abilities which are most likely related to their effects on monoamines in endogenous pain pathways. The efficacy of both serotonin and norepinephrine selective antidepressants would suggest that effects on pathways which involve either of these transmitters might contribute to analgesia. Other suggested mechanisms of analgesia involve the antihistamine properties of some agents, increased endorphin secretion, and an increased density of cortical calcium channels.[11, 56]

In a study of 44 patients admitted for low back pain, Jenkins et al. compared treatment with oral imipramine (Tofranil), 25 mg tid, with placebo over a four-week period. After treatment, no significant difference in improvement in straight leg raising, pain and stiffness assessments, nor psychological testing was noted between the two study groups. In those individuals with apparent discogenic pain, imipramine-treated patients demonstrated greater improvement in pain and stiffness, but this was not found to be statistically significant. No significant difference in side effects was noted between the two groups.[59] In a study of 48 patients with chronic low back pain, treatment with imipramine was compared to placebo. Seven of the patients included were determined clinically depressed according to standard criteria. Patients completed Beck depression questionnaires at both the initial and final visits. Depression score improvements, while not statistically significant, were noted in those patients who benefited from imipramine treatment. Individuals treated with imipramine did demonstrate a significant improvement in both limitations of work and restrictions in normal activities. Anticholinergic side effects were associated with a 10% dropout rate.[60]

In a review of the literature on antidepressants in the treatment of chronic low back pain, Egbunike et al. concluded that the most consistent responses were found with doxepin and desipramine at doses above 150 mg daily. Some studies may have failed to demonstrate a response secondary to inadequate dosing. Other antidepressants were found less effective in providing analgesia. In several studies reviewed, while improvements in depression were observed, poor correlations were noted between analgesic effects and changes in the severity of depression. The relationship between pain relief and antidepressant effect remains unclear.[61]

TCAs produce analgesia at lower dosages than are typically prescribed for the treatment of depression. The starting dose of the tricyclics should be low. Initial daily dosing of amitriptyline should be 10 mg in elderly patients and 25 mg in younger individuals. Every two to three days an increment in dosing equal to the initial starting dose can be made until adequate analgesia is achieved or adverse effects develop. The typical effective daily dose of amitriptyline ranges from 50 to 150 mg. As the TCA half-life is generally long and sedation is a common side effect, single nighttime dosing can be prescribed. Some patients report better pain relief and less morning drowsiness with divided daily dosing.[56, 11]

Studies that have investigated the analgesic efficacy of SSRIs have typically involved dosages similar to those prescribed in the management of depression, 20 to 40 mg of fluoxetine or paroxetine.[57, 62] Further research is needed in order to clarify the relationship between dosage and analgesia with the serotonin-specific agents.[56]

The occurrence of serious adverse effects resulting from antidepressant administration is low. These complications would be rare at the generally lower dosages utilized in the treatment of pain. While cardiac side effects are uncommon, tricyclics are contraindicated in those individuals with heart failure or serious cardiac conduction abnormalities. Orthostatic hypotension is the most frequent cardiovascular adverse effect, and the elderly are particularly at risk. The sedating effect often observed with antidepressant use can be beneficial as patients with pain often demonstrate diminished daytime functioning from inadequate sleep. Anticholinergic side effects such as dry mouth, blurred vision, and urinary retention are more likely with amitriptyline use than with other TCAs. These effects are also less likely at the lower dosages used for analgesia. Nortriptyline and desipramine have been found to induce fewer anticholinergic side effects and are less sedating.[11, 56]

While antidepressants have been demonstrated as useful adjuncts in the treatment of pain, their analgesic mechanism remains unclear. Initial dosing should be low and then slowly increased to minimize side effects. There appears to be a potential role for antidepressants in the treatment of the acute low back pain patient with pain and difficulties sleeping. When taken at night, the sedating properties of these agents can be beneficial in those pain patients experiencing difficulty with sleep.

7.7   Corticosteroids

The numerous effects of corticosteroids include: maintenance of fluid and electrolyte balance, alterations in carbohydrate, fat and protein metabolism, and preservation of the functions of the cardiovascular system and skeletal muscle. Prescribed corticosteroids are typically categorized according to their relative anti-inflammatory and sodium retaining potencies (Table 7.4). Steroid compounds are typically prescribed for their anti-inflammatory effects but often also display significant mineralocorticoid activity. Oral steroids have been found effective in the treatment of inflammatory reactions associated with allergic states, rheumatic and autoimmune diseases, and respiratory disorders. Corticosteroids interact with receptor proteins in target tissues to regulate gene expression and ultimately protein synthesis by the target tissue. As these interactions and regulatory processes occur slowly, most of the effects of corticosteroids are not immediate and become apparent hours following their introduction. Recent investigations have suggested an additional and more immediate component to corticosteroid action mediated by an interaction with membrane-bound protein receptors.[2, 48]

Over the past two decades, the biochemical contributions to sciatica and low back pain have been the focus of much attention.[49] In the late 1970s the nuclear material of the vertebral disc was found to be antigenic and capable of producing an in vitro autoimmune reaction. It was hypothesized that a chemical radiculitis might explain radicular pain in the absence of a more

Table 7.4

Steroid Compound	Anti-Inflammatory Potency	Sodium Retaining Potency	Biological Half-Life (Hours)	Equivalent Dose (mg)
Cortisol	1	1	8–12	20
Cortisone (Cortone)	0.8	0.8	8–12	25
Prednisone (Deltasone)	4	0.8	12–36	5
Prednisolone	4	0.8	12–36	5
6alpha-methyl prednisolone	5	0.5	12–36	4
Triamcinolone (Aristocort)	5	0	12–36	4
Dexamethasone (Decadron)	25	0	36–72	0.75

(1, 2)

mechanical stressor.[50] Phospholipase A2 (PLA2), a potent inflammatory mediator, has been demonstrated to be released by discs following injury.[51] The anti-inflammatory and immunosuppressive effects of glucocorticoids are largely secondary to their inhibition of the immune responses of lymphocytes, macrophages, and fibroblasts. Whereas NSAIDs principally inhibit prostaglandin synthesis, corticosteroids interfere earlier in the inflammatory cascade by inhibiting PLA2 actions and thereby curtailing both the leukotriene and prostaglandin mediated inflammatory response.[3]

Studies examining the use of oral steroids in the setting of acute low back pain are limited. In 1986, Haimovic and Beresford compared oral dexamethasone with placebo in the treatment of 33 patients with lumbosacral radicular pain. Subjects receiving dexamethasone were given a tapering dose, from 64 to 8 mg over seven days. Early improvements (within seven days) were not significantly different between the two groups, occurring in seven of 21 patients in the dexamethasone group and four of 12 in the placebo group. In those subjects initially found to have radicular type pain on straight leg-raising, however, eight of 19 treated with dexamethasone, compared with only one of six in the placebo group, had diminished pain on straight leg-raising repeated within seven days. The limitations of this study include a small subject number, the use of additional analgesics which may have obscured group differences, the clinical uncertainty of a radicular process in a significant number of subjects, and the loss of several patients to follow up after one year.[52]

In the setting of acute low back pain, oral corticosteroids are typically prescribed in a quick tapering fashion over one week. The biological half-lives differ among the steroid compounds (Table 7.4).

Multiple adverse effects have been associated with *prolonged* steroid use, including suppression of the hypothalamic-pituitary-adrenal axis, immunosuppression, pseudotumor cerebri and psychoses, cataracts and increased intraocular pressure, osteoporosis, avascular necrosis, gastric ulcers, fluid and electrolyte disturbances and hypertension, and impaired wound healing. The severity of these complications correlates with the dosage, duration of use, and the potency of the steroid prescribed. While the incidence of steroid induced myopathy does not appear to be directly related to the dosage of steroid prescribed nor the duration of use, it appears to be more prevalent with the use of steroids containing a 9-alpha fluorine configuration, such as triamcinolone. The relationship between hypertensive side effects and the duration of therapy is also not very clear; steroids should be prescribed with greater caution in the elderly, in those individuals with known hypertension, and when compounds with greater mineralocorticoid properties are prescribed. As hyperglycemia is a well-known complication of corticosteroid use, oral steroids should be prescribed with caution in the diabetic population.[53]

As potent anti-inflammatory agents, oral steroids represent a theoretically useful agent in the treatment of patients with radiculopathy due to local inflammation secondary to disc injury or herniation. While many adverse effects are associated with oral steroid use, these are more frequently encountered in the setting of prolonged administration. The effectiveness of oral steroids in the acute low back pain population remains unproven; further research in this area is needed.

7.8   Colchicine

While beneficial in the treatment of the crystal induced inflammation observed in gout and pseudogout, colchicine is only occasionally effective in the treatment of other types of arthritides.[2, 54] Colchicine has been regarded by some as the most powerful anti-inflammatory agent known to man.[54]

Over the past 30 years, Rask has treated thousands of patients with resistant disc disorders with oral and intravenous colchicine and has noted a 90–95% "improvement" rate. Since 1979, he has published the results of his uncontrolled studies, some involving up to 500 patients, which have suggested significant therapeutic benefits from colchicine therapy with fewer adverse effects than typically associated with the use of aspirin.[54, 55] In addition to colchicine's potent and anti-inflammatory abilities, other theories have been expounded in an attempt to explain its efficacy in the treatment of disc disease, including an inhibition of amyloidogenesis and an increase in endorphin production by the substantia gelatinosa.[54]

In a 1985 double-blind study of 39 patients with low back pain of at least two months' duration, Meek compared combined intravenous and oral colchicine treatment with placebo. Patients in the treatment group received colchicine 0.6 mg orally Bid for 14 days and one mg IV on Days 1, 4, and 8 of the 14-day study period. While no real effect from placebo administration was observed, the treatment group demonstrated significant improvements in pain, weakness, leg-raising limitations, and muscle spasm. Adverse effects from colchicine administration were documented in only one patient in the form of a burn at the IV site.[54] In a double-blind study of oral colchicine in the treatment of low back pain, Schnebel and Simmons compared oral colchicine with placebo in 34 patients with low back symptoms of less than three months duration. Over the 12-week study period, both groups of patients continued in a comprehensive physical therapy program and were administered NSAIDs and muscle relaxants. No significant differences in therapeutic response were noted between the treatment and placebo groups, but an increased number of adverse effects, mainly diarrhea and vomiting, were observed in the colchicine group. This study has several limitations, including a small sample size, multiple etiologies of low back pain, poor patient compliance, and the use of concomitant treatments.[55]

Colchicine use is contraindicated those patients with serious gastrointestinal renal, hepatic, or cardiac disease. Colchicine can also harm the fetus when used during pregnancy. When administered intravenously for the treatment of an acute gouty attack, the total dosage over the first 24 hours should not exceed 4 mg, as greater cumulative dosages have been associated with multiple organ failure and death.[3] Colchicine serves to inhibit the intracellular microtubules and mitotic spindles, and its adverse affects are largely secondary to its actions on the rapidly proliferating cells of the gastrointestinal epithelium. Abdominal pain, nausea, vomiting, and diarrhea, are typically the earliest and most common adverse effects associated with colchicine overdosage. These gastrointestinal side effects can be almost entirely avoided with intravenous use. Colchicine has also been noted to cause a transient leukopenia which is soon replaced with a leukocytosis. Myopathy and neuropathy have been noted in patients with impaired renal function receiving colchicine treatment.[3]

The use of colchicine in the treatment of the acute low back pain patient is not commonly practiced. While a few practitioners have found colchicine effective in this patient population, others have not. Further investigation in this area is needed before colchicine use can be recommended for the low back pain patient. These studies may be helpful in further defining colchicine's place among other available anti-inflammatory and analgesic agents.

7.9   Summary

There are various agents that can be helpful in addressing the painful phase of acute low back problems. The particular medication should be chosen after consideration of the following: indications; contraindications' goals of treatment, i.e., analgesia, reduction of inflammation, reduction of muscle spasm, etc.; and the scientific and clinical evidence demonstrating effectiveness. With the proper selection of pain medication effective pain relief can be used to progress the patient through the early phase of treatment and into an active exercise program.

7.10   References

1. Malanga, G. A. Medications in acute low back pain, in *Acute Low Back Pain,* Gonzales, E., ed. New York: Demos Vermande, New York, in press.
2. Hardman, J. G. and Limbird, L. E., eds. *Goodman and Gilman's The Pharmacological Basis of Therapeutics,* 9th ed.. New York: McGraw-Hill, 1996.
3. Westley, G. J., Schaefer, J., Sifton, D. W., eds. *Physicians' Desk Reference,* 49th ed. Montvale NJ: Medical Economics, 1995.
4. Amadio, P. Jr. and Cummings, D. M. Evaluation of acetaminophen in the management of osteoarthritis of the knee. *Curr. Ther. Res.* 34:59–66, 1983.
5. Doyle, D. V. and Lanham, J. G. Routine drug treatment of osteoarthritis. *Clin. Rheumatol. Dis.* 10:277–91, 1984.
6. Calin, A. Pain and inflammation. *Am. J. Med.* 77:Suppl 3A:9–15, 1984.
7. Bradley, J. D., Brandt, K. D., Katz, B. P., Kalasinski, L. A., and Ryan, S. I. Comparison of an anti-inflammatory dose of ibuprofen, an analgesic dose of

ibuprofen, and acetaminophen in the treatment of patients with osteoarthritis of the knee. *New Eng. J. Med.* 325:87–91, 1991.

8.   Hickey, R. F. J. Chronic low back pain: a comparison of diflunisal with paracetamol. *New Zeal. Med. J.* 95:312–14, 1982.

9.   Brooks, P. M. and Day, R. O. Nonsteroidal anti-inflammatory drugs — differences and similarities. *New Engl. J. Med.* 324:1716–25, 1991.

10. Weiler, J. M. The use of nonsteroidal antiinflammatory drugs (NSAIDs) in sports soft-tissue injury. *Clin. Sports Med.* 11:625–44, 1992.

11. Portenoy, R. K. and Kanner, R. M., eds. *Pain Management: Theory and Practice.* Philadelphia: F. A. Davis, 1996.

12. Abramowicz, M. ed. Drugs for pain. *The Med. Lett.* 35:1–6, 1993.

13. McCormack, K. and Brune, K. Dissociation between the antinociceptive and anti-inflammatory effects of the non-steroidal anti-inflammatory drugs. *Drugs* 41:533–47, 1991.

14. Malmerg, A. B. and Yaksh, T. L. Hyperalgesia mediated by spinal glutamate or substance receptor blocked by spinal cyclooxygenase inhibition. *Science* 257:1276–79, 1992.

15. Gebhart, G. F. and McCormack, K. J. Neuronal plasticity. Implication for pain therapy. *Drugs* 47 Suppl. 5:1–47, 1994.

16. Konttinen, Y. T., Kemppinen, P., Segerberg, M., Hukkanen, M., Recs, R., Santavirta, S., Sorsa, T., Pertovaara, A., and Polak, J. M. Peripheral and spinal neural mechanisms in arthritis with particular reference to treatment of inflammation and pain. *Arthrit. Rheum.* 37:965–82, 1994.

17. Gaucher, A., Netter, P., Faure, G., Schoeller, J. P., and Gerardin, A. Diffusion of oxyphenbutazone into synovial fluid, synovial tissue, joint cartilage and cerebrospinal fluid. *Eur. J. Clin. Pharm.* 25:107–12, 1983.

18. McCormack, K. and Brune, K. Toward defining the analgesic role of nonsteroidal anti-inflammatory drugs in the management of acute soft tissue injuries. *Clin. J. Sports Med.* 3:106–17, 1993.

19. Amlie, E., Weber, H. and Holme, I. Treatment of acute low back pain with piroxicam: results of a double-blind placebo-controlled trial. *Spine* 12(5):473–6, 1987.

20. Wasner, C., Britton, M. C., Kraines, R. G., Kaye, R. L., Bobrove, A. M., and Fries, J. F. Nonsteroidal antiinflammatory agents in rheumatoid arthritis and ankylosing spondylitis. *JAMA* 246(19):2168–72, 1981.

21. Hayllar, J. and Bjarnason, I. NSAIDs, COX-2 inhibitors, and the gut (commentary). *Lancet* 346:521–2, 1995.

22. Jiranek, G. C., Kimmey, M. B., Saunders, D. R., Willson, R. A., Shanahan, W., and Silverstein, F. E. Misoprostol reduces gastrointestinal injury from one week of aspirin: An endoscopic study. *Gastroenterology* 96:656–61, 1989.

23. Radford, M. G., Holley, K. E., Grande, J. P., Larson, T. S., Wagoner, R. D., Donadio, J., and McCarthy, J. T. Reversible membranous nephropathy associated with use of nonsteroidal anti-inflammatory drugs. *JAMA* 276(6):466–69, 1996.

24. Buckwalter, J. A. Current concepts review. Pharmacological treatment of soft-tissue injuries. *J. Bone Jt. Surg.* 77A(12):1902–14, 1995.

25. Almekinders, L. C., Baynes, A. J. and Bracey L. W. An in vitro investigation into the effects of repetitive motion and nonsteroidal antiinflammatory medication on human tendon fibroblasts. *Am. J. Sports Med.* 23(4):119–23, 1995.

26. Almekinders, L. C. and Gilbert, J. A. Healing of experimental muscle strains an the effects of nonsteroidal anti-inflammatory medication. *Am. J. Sports Med.* 14(4):303–308, 1986.

27. Mishra, D. K., Friden, J., Schmitz, M. C., and Lieber, R. L. Anti-inflammatory medication after muscle injury. *J. Bone Jt. Surg.* 77A(10):1510–19, 1995.

28. De Lee, J. C. and Rockwood, C. A. Skeletal muscle spasm and a review of muscle relaxants. *Curr. Ther. Res.*, 27(4):64–73, 1980.

29. Rollings, H. E., Glassman, J. M. and Soyka, J. P. Management of acute musculoskeletal conditions-thoracolumbar strain or sprain: a double-blind evaluation comparing the efficacy and safety of carisoprodol with cyclobenzaprine hydrochloride. *Curr. Ther. Res.* 34(6):917–27, 1983.

30. Hindle, T. H. Comparison of carisoprodol, butabarbital, and placebo in the treatment of the low back syndrome. *Calif. Med.* 117:7–11, 1972.

31. Basmajian, J. V. Acute low back pain and spasm. A controlled multicenter trial of combined analgesic and antispasm agents. *Spine* 14(4):438–9, 1989.

32. Borenstein, D. G., Lacks, S., Wiesel, S. W. Cyclobenzaprine and naproxen versus naproxen alone in the treatment of acute low back pain and muscle spasm. *Clin. Ther.* 12(4):125–31, 1990.

33. Baratta, R. R. A double-blind study of cyclobenzaprine and placebo in the treatment of acute musculoskeletal conditions of the low back. *Curr. Ther. Res.* 32(5):646–52, 1982.

34. Hingorani, K. Diazepam in backache. A double-blind controlled trial. *Ann Phys Med* 8:303–6, 1965.

35. Boyles, W. F., Glassman, J. M. and Soyka, J. P. Management of acute musculoskeletal conditions: Thoracolumbar strain or sprain. *Tod. Ther. Trends* 1:1–16, 1983.

36. Casale, R. Acute low back pain. Symptomatic treatment with a muscle relaxant drug. *The Clin. J. Pain.* 4:81–88, 1988.

37. Daoas, F., Hartman, S. E., Martinez, L., Northrup, B. E., Nussodorf, T., Silberman, H. M., and Gross, H. Baclofen for the treatment of acute low back syndrome. A double-blind comparison with placebo. *Spine* 10(4):345–49, 1985.

38. Brown, F. L., Bodison, S., Dixon, J., Davis, W., and Nowoslawski, J. Comparison of diflunisal and acetaminophen with codeine in the treatment of initial or recurrent low back strain. *Clin. Ther.* 9(Supp C):1986.

39. Wiesel, S. W., Cuckler, J. M., Deluca, F., Jones, F., Zeide, M. S., and Rothman, R. H. Acute low back pain. An objective analysis of conservative therapy. *Spine* 4:324–30, 1980.

40. Cooper, S. A., Engel, J., Ladove, M., Rauch, D., Precheur, H., and Rosenheck, A. An evaluation of oxycodone and acetaminophen in the treatment of postoperative dental pain. *Clin. Pharm. Ther.* 25(4):219, 1979.

41. Hopkinson, J. H., Bartlett, F. H., Steffens, A. O., McGlumphy, T. H., Macht, E. L., and Smith, M. Acetaminophen versus propoxyphene hydrochloride for relief of pain in episiotomy patients. *J. Clin. Phar.* 13:251–63, 1973.

42. Wilder-Smith, C. H., Schimke, J., Osterwalder, B., and Senn, H. J. Oral tramadol, a mu-opioid agonist and monoamine reuptake-blocker, and morphine for strong cancer related pain. *Ann. Oncol.* 5(4):141–6, 1994.

43. Sunshine, A., Olson, N. Z., Zighelboim, I., DeCastro, A., and Minn, F. L. Analgesic oral efficacy of tramadol hydrochloride in postoperative pain. *Clin. Pharm. Ther.* 51(6):740–6, 1992.

44. Rauk, R. L., Ruoff, G. E., and McMillen, J. I. Comparison of tramadol and aceta-minophen with codeine for long-term pain management in elderly patients. *Curr. Ther. Res.* 55(12):1417–31, 1994.

45. Preston, K. L., Jasinski, D. R., and Testa, M. Abuse potential and pharmacological comparison of tramadol and morphine. *Drug. Alch. Dep.* 27(4):7–17, 1991.

46. Houmes, R. J., Voets, M. A., Verkaaik, A., Erdmann, W., and Lachmann, B. Efficacy and safety of tramadol versus morphine for moderate and severe postoperative pain with special regard to respiratory depression. *Anesth. Analg.* 74(4):510–4, 1992.

47. Kaiko, R. F., Foley, K. M., Grabinski, P. Y. et al. Central nervous system excitatory effects of meperidine in cancer patients. *Ann. Neur.* 13:180–5, 1983.

48. Wehlig, M. Novel aldosterone receptors: specificity conferring mechanism at the level of the cell membrane. *Steroids* 59:160–3, 1994.

49. Nicholas, J. A. and Hershman, E. B., eds. *The Lower Extremity and Spine in Sports Medicine.* vol. II. St. Louis: Mosby, 1995.

50. Marshall, L. L., Trethewie, E. R., and Curtain, C. C. Chemical radiculitis: a clinical, physiological and immunological study. *Clin. Orthop.* 129:61, 1979.

51. Saal J. S. et al. High levels of phospholipase A2 activity in lumbar spine disc herniation. *Spine* 15:164, 1990.

52. Haimovic, I. C. and Beresford, H. R. Dexamethasone is not superior to placebo for treating lumbosacral radicular pain. *Neurology* 36:1593–94, 1986.

53. Truhan, A. P. and Ahmed, A. R. Corticosteroids: a review with emphasis on complications of prolonged systemic therapy. *Ann. of Allerg.* 62:375–90, 1989.

54. Meek, J. B., Giudice, V. W., McFadden, J. W., Key, J. D., and Enrick, N. L. Colchicine confirmed as highly effective in disk disorders. Final results of a double blind study. *J. Neur. Orth. Med. Surg.* 6(4):211–18, 1985.

55. Schnebel, B. E. and Simmons, J. W. The use of oral colchicine for low back pain. A double-blind study. *Spine* 13(4):354–57, 1988.

56. King, S. A. Antidepressants: A valuable adjunct for musculoskeletal pain. *J. Musculoskel. Med.* October:51–57, 1995.

57. Magni, G. The use of antidepressants in the treatment of chronic pain. A review of the current evidence. *Drugs* 42:730–48, 1991.

58. Jacox, A., Carr, D. B., Payne, R. et al. Management of cancer pain. Clinical practice guideline no. 9. Rockville, MD: Agency for Health Care Policy and Research; 1994. U.S. Dept. of Health and Human Services, Public Health Service, AHCPR Publication No. 94-0592.

59. Jenkins, D. G., Ebbut, A. F. and Evans, C. D. Tofranil in the treatment of low back pain. *J. Int. Med. Res.* 4(Supp 2):28–40, 1976.

60. Alcoff, J., Jones, E., Rust, P. and Newman, R. Controlled trial of imipramine for chronic low back pain. *J. Fam. Pract.* 14(5):841–6, 1982.

61. Egbunike, I. G. and Chaffee, B. J. Antidepressants in the management of chronic pain syndromes. *Pharmacother.* 10(4):262–70, 1990.

62. Max, M. B., Lynch, S. A., Muir, J. et al. Effects of desipramine, amitriptyline, and fluoxetine on pain in diabetic neuropathy. *N. Eng. J. Med.* 326:1250–56, 1992.

63. Abramowicz, ed. Drugs for rheumatoid arthritis. *Med. Lett.* 36:101–6, 1994.

64. American Pain Society. Principles of Analgesic Use in the Treatment of Acute Pain and Cancer Pain. (3rd ed.). Skokie, IL: 1993.

chapter eight

Therapeutic Injections for Low Back Pain

Mark V. Reecer, M.D.
Jeffrey L. Woodward, M.D., M.S.

8.1   Overview

In order for a patient to participate fully in a comprehensive rehabilitation program, the cause of their low back pain needs to be identified and treated appropriately. There are several therapeutic injection procedures which are available to reduce pain and augment the use of conservative measures to improve the patient's functional status. If patients do not respond to initial conservative measures, therapeutic injections can be considered. Specific injection techniques and locations will be dependent upon the patient's history, physical examination, and diagnostic studies. The relief from some injection procedures may be temporary; however, with reduction in pain inhibition, patients can assume a more active role in their rehabilitation program.

8.2   Epidural Steroid Injections

Therapeutic lumbar epidural steroid injections (LESI) traditionally have involved the injection of corticosteroid to provide pain relief from active inflammation involving lumbar epidural tissues and adjacent neural structures. While most prior outcome studies of therapeutic epidural steroid injections have usually indicated temporary pain relief only, some patients may experience significant lasting relief reducing the need for other treatments. In addition, there are several potential clinical benefits for time-limited pain relief as well. Some of these benefits would include an opportunity for the patient to progress: physical activity and more formal therapy and exercise programs; the time period of reduced pain during which medications may be significantly reduced, including nonsteroidal anti-inflammatories and narcotic analgesics; and an increased sense of confidence on the part of the patient that the treating physician has properly diagnosed the site of active injury and pain.

While there may be some brief pain relief following the epidural injection of local anesthetics, possibly due to both the physical effects of the fluid itself on inflamed tissues, as well as the interruption of afferent nerve impulses decreasing the level of pain,[23] longer duration pain relief is more commonly noted following use of injectates containing corticosteroids. The pain relieving effect of steroids have become more understandable as the role of the inflammatory cascade and phospholipase A2 levels have become more clearly understood.[80, 90, 100] The primary mechanism of action of epidural corticosteroid continues to be attributed mainly to the anti-inflammatory properties of the steroid solution.[40, 106] A study by Winnie demonstrated the pain-relieving potential of corticosteroid by noting significant back and leg pain relief responses following epidural injection of only 2 ml of corticosteroids with no other components.[112] More recently, Lee et al. has reported an animal model finding of radiculopathy associated with increased levels of phospholipase A2 activity initiated by local inflammation of the nerve root and a subsequent decrease of the phospholipase A2 chemical activity following the administration of local corticosteroid solution.[75] Radicular pain relief following epidural corticosteroid injection may also be due to the stabilization of nerve root membranes through corticosteroid suppression of ectopic neuronal discharges which can cause pain and paresthesias.[26, 105]

Several literature reviews of pertinent outcome studies evaluating the pain relieving effect of LESI for both the low back and radicular pain have been published recently.[113, 114] Evaluation of epidural outcome studies reveals that most of the prior lumbar epidural steroid injection clinical studies have been relatively poorly randomized and controlled. The published response rate indicating the percentage of patients having significant pain relief following epidural steroid injection has been reported from a low of 20% to a high of 100%.[15, 67] In thorough reviews, Kepes and Duncalf indicated an average lumbar epidural steroid response rate of 60% and White et al. reported an average of 75% of treated patients noting significant pain relief.[107] Three meta-analysis studies of prior LESI outcome data have been published prior to Carrette's study,[21] and although meta-analysis results are only as good as the data which is available to analyze, these statistical techniques do help to increase the power of the available data by combining the results of numerous studies. Rapp, Haselcorn, and Elam reported meta-analysis results in 1994 on LESI which revealed a modest but significant pain relief benefit from lumbar epidural steroids for both low back and radicular pain.[88] Watts and Silagy in 1995 combined the results of 11 Australian LESI trials for their meta-analysis study.[104] Their report indicated that patients having significant radicular pain were 2.6 to 3 times more likely to have at least 75% back and leg pain relief up to 60 days following the injection as compared to placebo treatment. Study patients were also two times more likely to have significantly decreased back and leg pain 12 months following epidural steroid injection versus placebo treatment. These authors indicated that their study provided quantitative evidence supporting the efficacy of epidural steroids radicularly for the treatment of radicular pain. Carrette did demonstrate short-term benefit of corticosteroid injections in the first six weeks, which can promote active participation in a comprehensive rehabilitation program. There was no long-term benefit of the injections when comparing the placebo and injection group three months after the procedure.[21]

From the various reviews of epidural steroid injection responses for both back and radicular pain, some general trends have become evident. Typically, the best pain relief results are noted for steroid injections performed on patients having radicular pain for up to three months' duration with chronic back and radicular pain having less reliable relief.[52, 61] Better pain relief responses were also noted from epidural steroids performed on patients having pain directly associated with acute disc injury and pathology.[52, 107] Substantial pain relief is more likely to occur for LESI with radicular pain as compared with only paraspinal or axial pain.[107] Also, post-surgical patients tend to have less pain relief from LESI unless an acute recurrent disc herniation or recent onset of acute radiculopathy is present. Most commonly, the pain relief reported in clinical trials following epidural steroid injection typically began within a few days to a week following the steroid injection and the duration of statistically significant pain relief tended to last up to, but no more than, several months' time.[63, 107] Specifically, White et al. reported 82% of patients having pain relief duration of one day after LESI, 24% with pain relief one month postinjection, 16% after two months, and 7% with pain relief for at least six months postinjection. One prior study has indicated that the long-term functional status of patients improved following epidural steroid injection compared to controlled patients with respect to decreased return-to-work time following injury.[28]

Patient selection guidelines for administering LESI have yet to be clearly established through clinical testing or by consensus agreement of spine injectionists. Certainly, some of the general trends in LESI response just reviewed can be used to improve patient selection and clinical outcomes. Commonly, patients are provided at least some initial period of time for gradual pain relief for acute low back or radicular pain with time for rest and recovery as well as with basic conservative care prior to considering LESI. If a patient is managing the back and/or leg pain adequately, then a minimum of three to six weeks' time prior to considering LESI may be appropriate since many patients with less severe injuries will have significant clinical recovery within this time period. However, in our opinion, it is not medically unreasonable to consider LESI particularly for severe unremitting radicular pain after a period of time of even one to two weeks, depending on the patient's clinical status and narcotic analgesic usage and effect. The patients requiring routine consideration for initial LESI are those having symptoms indicative of either discogenic and/or radicular pain. An experienced physician does not need a lumbar CT or MRI scan prior to the initial LESI which can be done safely and effectively strictly based on clinical judgment.[48] No clear clinical rationale exists for performing a series of three LESIs at predetermined intervals since positive pain responses may often last four to eight weeks from a single injection and some patients with acute lumbar or radicular pain may recover adequately after receiving only one or two injections. It is generally accepted that if the initial epidural steroid injection provides absolutely no relief, then repeat injections, particularly injections performed at the identical injection site, are not recommended.[7, 12, 62] From our prior review of the epidural steroid injection literature, it is traditionally recommended that a total of three LESI's maximum be performed within 12 months' time due to the possible cumulative side effects of corticosteroid injection. Stambaugh recommended the following absolute contraindications for LESI: (1) cauda equina syndrome; (2) anticoagulation or bleeding disorders; and (3) suspected local or systemic infection.[99]

The choice of the specific approach and needle location within the lumbar spine for LESI depends on several factors including the pathoanatomy (e.g., lateral versus central disc herniation), intrinsic anatomic factors (e.g., the presence of a spinal fusion), and response to any previous injections. The various approaches to the epidural space include caudal, translaminar, and transforaminal epidural injections. A general principle to follow for placement of the corticosteroid injectate is to perform the approach allowing steroid infiltration as close as possible to the suspected source of pathology and pain. Caudal epidural injections (Figures 8.1 and 8.2) are effective for sacral and L5 radiculopathies. More cephalad flow of medication for higher lumbar radiculopathies is unreliable though. The use of caudal epidurals offers advantages including the bilateral and anterior and posterior flow of medication, and a lower risk of dural puncture.

Patients having primarily lumbar, gluteal, and proximal thigh discomfort only with discogenic characteristics can often be treated effectively with a posterior translaminar (Figure 8.3) or transflaval needle approach.

More recently, transforaminal approaches to the epidural space have been touted as a means of placing the steroid solution more selectively to a single spine level and at the anterior epidural space along posterior annular tissue. Patients having clear and specific radicular pain consistent with a single dermatomal pattern, and especially those having much more significant leg versus lumbar pain, are often more effectively treated with selective nerve root steroid injection. Selective nerve root injection involves advancing the needle tip closely adjacent to the neural tissue and injecting corticosteroid only after obtaining a fluoroscopic neurogram indicating needle placement within the epiradicular membrane of that nerve root. A recent study indicates that lumbar epidural perineural steroid injection is more effective in the

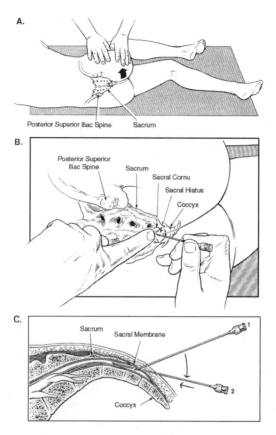

Figure 8.1 Caudal epidural injection. From Willis, R. Caudal epidural blockade, in *Neural Blockade in Clinical Anesthesia and Management of Pain*, 2nd ed., Cousins, M. J., Bridenbaugh, P. O. eds. New York: J. B. Lippincott Co., 1988, with permission.

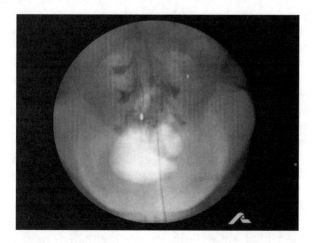

Figure 8.2 Caudal epidural injection with contrast under fluoroscopy.

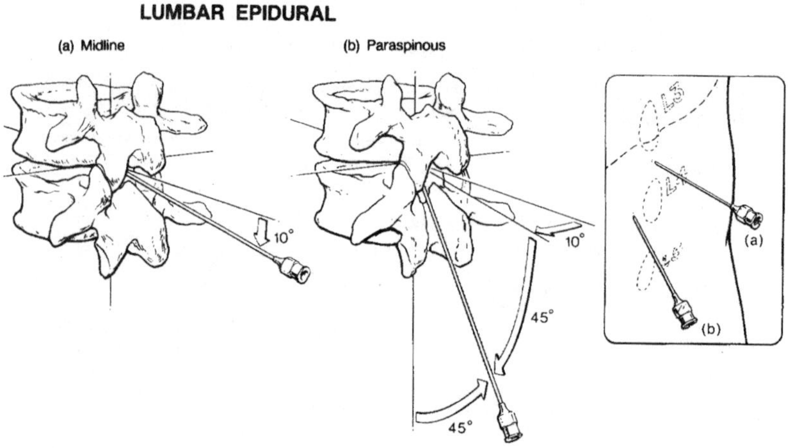

LUMBAR EPIDURAL

Figure 8.3 Translaminar epidural injection techniques using midline (a) and paraspinous (b) approaches. From Cousins, M.J., Bromage, P.R. Epidural neural blockade, in *Neural Blockade in Clinical Anesthesia and Management of Pain, 2nd ed.*, Cousins, M.J., Bridenbaugh P.O. eds., New York: J.B. Lippincott Co., 1988, with permission.

relief of lower extremity radicular pain as compared to the more traditional posterior translaminar epidural steroid injection approach.[71] Translaminar or transflaval epidural steroid injections typically should not be performed at spinal levels at which previous laminectomy surgical procedures have been performed. Since laminectomy/discectomy procedures may have completely obliterated the epidural space with fibrosis, the risk of dural puncture during an attempted epidural injection usually becomes unacceptable. However, careful placement of a 25-gauge spinal needle, particularly in the lateral epidural space for significant post-surgical back and radicular pain, can be attempted at the patient's and the physician's risk. For postsurgical patients, a transforaminal approach is most recommended and safe (Figure 8.4), although foraminal fibrosis can interfere with the free flow of injectate into the spinal canal.

Various corticosteroid preparations are available for epidural steroid injections, with the most common preparations being betamethasone, methylprednisolone acetate, and triamcinolone diacetate. The authors recommend the use of the commercially available steroid solution, Celestone Soluspan. This particular corticosteroid solution is comprised of a mixture of betamethasone sodium phosphate and betamethasone acetate, with the former being highly soluble and fast acting within minutes to hours and the latter component existing as a microfine particle suspended in the liquid vehicle with relatively slow absorption and a longer duration of action. Celestone Soluspan is also clinically indicated because of the absence of any harmful preservatives present in this particular steroid mixture. Numerous adverse side effects from LESI are well-documented, although most are brief and

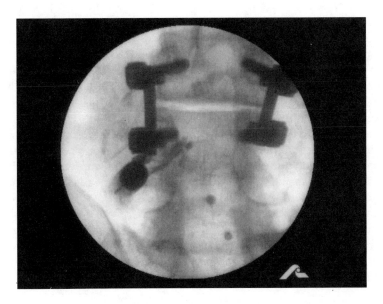

Figure 8.4   Transforaminal injection in patient with prior instrumented lumbar fusion.

well-tolerated. The most common short-term side effects reported by patients following epidural administration of glucocorticoid steroids reported by Andrade include insomnia (39%), facial flushing (29%), nausea (21%), itching (21%), fever described as "feeling hot" with temperature <100 degrees (10%), and rash (8%). A small number of patients reported nonpositional headaches, anxiousness, elevated blood pressure, dizziness and "weakness."[2] Longer duration and potentially more serious side effects from LESI can be caused by significant depression of plasma cortisol levels following steroid injection. The depression of normal cortisol levels can continue for several weeks following LESI as previously documented for epidural methylprednisolone.[19] One prior case report indicated significantly decreased cortisol levels and chronic suppression of ACTH secretion occurring after a total of three triamcinolone LESIs done at weekly intervals.[87] There have also been several case reports of iatrogenically induced Cushing's syndrome secondary to either repeat or excessive dosage epidural steroid injections.[70, 103] Typically, however, LESI's are relatively safe procedures when done judiciously with Brown reporting no serious side effects in 500 LESI patients,[18] and White quoting a rate of significant complications at 0.4% following LESI in 300 patients.[106] Diabetics should be warned of the hyperglycemic properties of corticosteroids and typically a daily check of serum glucose should be performed for seven days following LESI and appropriate adjustment of diabetic medications provided for proper management of the transient hyperglycemia. In the author's experience, limiting the volume of Celestone Soluspan injected with any single epidural injection to 2.5 ml (approximately equivalent potency to a dose of methylprednisolone 80 mg) will satisfactorily limit the potential adverse reactions of the steroid while still providing reliable and effective clinical results. Any corticosteroid solution injected into the epidural space may cause a temporary increase in pain lasting 48 to 72 hours following the injection presumably due to chemical irritation from the steroid and possibly pain from increased hydrostatic pressure on inflamed epidural tissue immediately following the injection.[5, 24]

Fluoroscopy is recommended for all lumbar epidural steroid procedures in order to reduce potential complications from inadvertent intrathecal or intravascular injection and increase the response rate as much as possible from accurate needle placement. It has been reported that the rate of incorrect needle placement without the use of fluoroscopy is 13–30%.[32] Obviously, certain epidural approaches absolutely cannot be performed properly without fluoroscopic guidance due to anatomic considerations (such as selective nerve root injections); however, even translaminar or transflaval posterior approach epidural injections are best performed under fluoroscopic guidance for best results.[113, 114]

8.3   Facet Joint Injections

Therapeutic lumbar facet or zygapophyseal joint (Z-joint) procedures include intra-articular corticosteroid injection and medial branch of dorsal ramus (MBDR) neurolysis procedures with either chemical or radiofrequency nerve ablation. These procedures are intended to provide a longer duration pain relief from low back discomfort originating from within the Z-joint or from the surrounding joint capsule as opposed to the brief, but diagnostic, relief from the previously reviewed Z-joint diagnostic procedures. Detailed review of the prevalence of lumbar Z-joint pain is also contained in the previous diagnostic Z-joint chapter in this textbook. Prior research has indicated that lumbar Z-joint pain is a verifiable source of both acute and chronic low back pain, although the likelihood of patients having active Z-joint pain seems to vary considerably between various patient populations.[91] Although it could be argued that Z-joint anesthetic blockage via either intra-articular or MBDR nerve anesthesia may have at least some brief therapeutic effect, possibly through temporary interruption of nociceptive neural activity, therapeutic Z-joint treatment would commonly include only corticosteroid injection or a denervation procedure. Before considering a Z-joint ablative procedure for a patient, however, it is strongly recommended that prior diagnosis of active Z-joint lumbar pain should be confirmed with preferably two successful diagnostic Z-joint blocks.[11, 30] Another important tenet regarding the proper use of therapeutic Z-joint injections is the practice of using these procedures only as a part of a more diverse and comprehensive treatment program including therapeutic manual and exercise therapies.[34]

Numerous clinical studies are published in the literature regarding the efficacy of the various Z-joint therapeutic injection procedures, although the majority of these studies are poorly controlled designs and do not meet the accepted standards required to provide a strict randomized controlled treatment trial.[30] Uncontrolled studies of intra-articular Z-joint steroid injections have been associated with inconsistent therapeutic benefit with regard to pain relief as noted in prior published literature reviews.[31] The Dreyer et al. review did report long-term pain relief response greater than six months in uncontrolled studies of intra-articular Z-joint injections ranging from 18% to 63% of total patients treated.[31] Carette et al. did compare intra-articular steroid Z-joint injection with other Z-joint pain treatments.[22] Although this study was not a fully randomized controlled trial and patients receiving co-intervention were excluded, the authors did document that 46% of patients injected with methylprednisolone into lumbar Z-joints reported six months of marked pain relief, at least indicating the potential for significant long-term relief resulting from these injections. Lilius et al. performed lumbar intra-articular Z-joint injections and studied three experimental groups including a steroid-only group, a saline-only group, and a periarticular steroid with anesthetic group.[76] The authors indicated that overall 36% of patients reported significant pain relief for at least three months without a statistically significant difference between the saline only and the intra-articular steroid group. They indicated that, due to those results, specific therapeutic benefit from corticosteroid Z-joint injection was in question. However, Lynch and Taylor reported a statistically significant greater pain relief outcome from Z-joint intra-articular steroid without any local anesthetic included versus extra-articular Z-joint injection, with all of the injections being performed under fluoroscopy.[79] Of note, many of the prior Z-joint therapeutic injection experimental trials did not include confirmation of lumbar Z-joint pain as the correct diagnosis with diagnostic blocks prior to the therapeutic injections confusing the interpretation of the results since nonresponders to those therapeutic Z-joint injections may not have obtained significant pain relief from the procedure due to the absence of active Z-joint pain all along. Dreyer and Dreyfuss did report that some prior Z-joint studies revealed better pain response in patients with radiographic Z-joint degenerative changes as compared to the response in patients with no radiographic Z-joint arthropathy. Other studies have indicated better long-term relief in patients without Z-joint radiographic abnormality.[30]

In summary, discrepancies do exist between the conclusions of the various published outcome studies of therapeutic Z-joint injections. However, a number of prior studies do confirm the potential for significant and prolonged pain relief from therapeutic Z-joint procedures, suggesting that these relatively safe procedures should be considered when appropriate. It has been presumed that the primary pain-relieving effect of intra-articular corticosteroid injections is due to do the well-established anti-inflammatory effects of the steroid solution. Therapeutic corticosteroid Z-joint injections involve injecting a total of 1.0–2.0 ml total solution volume directly into the Z-joint with at least 50% of the injectate volume comprised of steroid and the remaining volume of concentrated local anesthetic such as 2% to 4% lidocaine or 0.5% to 0.75% marcaine. If active Z-joint pain has already been established with diagnostic blocks, then the entire volume of injectate can be steroid. Several corticosteroid preparations have been used in the past for these injections, although we would recommend Celestone Soluspan (containing a mixture of two betamethasone steroid ingredients) due to the presence of both short- and long-acting components and a relative lack of risk of crystalline precipitants following injection. If two to four lumbar Z-joints are injected at one time with corticosteroid following strict intra-articular injection protocol, there is typically no detectable systemic corticosteroid effect or risk due to that limited volume of injectate required. Corticosteroid Z-joint injection can be performed at any time after diagnosis of active Z-joint pain is made by diagnostic procedures. Typically, steroid Z-joint injections would not be done initially for acute back pain until at least four to six weeks' time for recovery and other treatments were tried and failed. Intra-articular Z-joint steroid injection could conceivably be repeated numerous times if reasonably prolonged and significant pain relief was noted. However, the cumulative deleterious effect of intra-articular corticosteroid on joint cartilage has been proposed in various peripheral joints and intuitively the risk for such intra-articular damage exists within Z-joint steroid injection in these weight-bearing joints.[51] It would seem pertinent then to limit the number of specific Z-joint steroid injections to three times yearly within the same joint and the total number to perhaps six to eight injections within any one Z-joint. If the first two to three intra-articular steroid injections all work adequately, then more long-lasting or possibly even permanent relief via MBDR denervation procedures for the Z-joint pain should be strongly considered.

The specific procedural technique used to perform intra-articular lumbar Z-joint steroid injection is identical to the intra-articular injection technique described in the previous diagnostic injection section of this text. The clinical pain response to a Z-joint steroid injection usually occurs within three to seven days following the injection. MBDR denervation procedures should not be considered or performed until after at least two successful diagnostic anesthetic MBDR injections have been performed. The basic techniques for MBDR neuroablation injections were described initially by Shealy in 1975.[93] Bogduk has subsequently detailed lumbar Z-joint neuroanatomy and the related MBDR injection techniques.[11] Due to the associated risk and discomfort of Z-joint denervation procedures, these procedures are usually reserved for patients having a more chronic duration of Z-joint pain, such as greater than six months, and patients who have failed to respond to multiple prior treatment modalities.[109] Windsor and Dreyer reviewed the results of eleven previous reports on lumbar Z-joint denervation treatments.[109] These authors state that in patients without prior lumbar surgery, the reviews indicate 60% to 80% of patients having good to excellent pain relief following Z-joint denervation procedure. The success rate for these procedures in patients with prior lumbar surgery without fusion is noted to be approximately 30% to 60%, and only about 30% of patients obtain prolonged good to excellent pain relief from the MBDR denervation procedure following prior lumbar fusion surgery. Other studies have also reiterated the trend that MBDR denervation procedures provide more reliable and long-term pain relief in patients without any prior lumbar surgery.[30, 92]

The specific procedural techniques for placing the needle for MBDR nerve injection have been described in the diagnostic section of this textbook. MBDR denervation may be accomplished with either the injection of phenol, a potent chemical neurolytic, or glycerin. Heat denaturation of these nerve fibers can be performed via radiofrequency techniques or cryoablation. Appropriate precautions must be taken when injecting phenol for MDBR ablation, including eye protection for all of those individuals working with the patient as well as skin protection, including protective garments and gloves due to the caustic nature of phenol. Most references recommend the use of 5% to 10% phenol solution, although in our experience using at least 7% solution is necessary. Due to the relative thick consistency of most phenol solutions, it is usually required that either a 22-gauge or even an 18-gauge spinal needle be used to perform MBDR phenol injection. No more than 1.0 ml phenol should be injected at any single transverse process injection site and the injection should be performed slowly following strict needle placement guidelines to avoid as much risk as possible from the phenol injection, particularly nerve root injury. Dreyfuss injects 80% glycerin using a 22-gauge needle. Due to the viscosity of the glycerin, there is minimal spread using a 22-gauge needle, allowing it to remain target specific. MBDR neuroablation using radiofrequency probe has become gradually more common over the past decade. The authors are unaware of any controlled studies that would indicate a significant difference between chemical versus radiofrequency MBDR denervation results. Gallagher published the only double-blind, randomized trial on radiofrequency ablation. Although the methods were somewhat suspect, the study did show benefit from the radiofrequency ablation procedure.[47] A thorough description of the proper use and technique for radiofrequency MBDR denervation is presented by Windsor and Dreyer in another recent textbook.[109] Strict adherence to the procedure techniques is necessary to reduce the risk of inadvertent injury to surrounding structures. There are no reports on denervation of the multifious muscles causing destabilization of that segment or accelerating degenerative disc changes.

8.4 Trigger Point Injections

Soft tissue injury is a very common cause of lower back pain. The areas of tenderness may present as highly localized, exquisitely sensitive areas and bands of skeletal muscle fibers. These areas are referred to as trigger points. With activation, these trigger points produce localized pain as well as referred pain in a myotomal pattern. Attempts have been made to quantitate and measure the presence of myofascial trigger points; however, consistent assessment of trigger points has been found to be unreliable. Typically these areas are tender to pressure and have palpable areas of hard resistance in the tissue which is felt to be a group of the affected muscle fibers in constant contraction.[39] It is important to remember that trigger points and zygapophysial joint pain can have remarkably similar pain distributions. This is due to the overlapping segmental nerve supply. A trigger point and/or facet joint can activate a segmental nerve with resultant concordant pain referral patterns.[13]

Modalities, stretching, and exercise can be used to manage trigger points; however, needling has been demonstrated to be the most effective treatment.[39] Local anesthetics can provide temporary pain relief; however, it appears that the long-term relief from the pain is actually from the mechanical disruption of the affected tissue and interruption of the trigger point mechanism.[45]

There are multiple injection techniques which have been described.[64, 101] Fischer has reported the most effective technique being a combination of needling with infiltration of 1% lidocaine or 0.5% procaine. Steroids have not been proven to be essential for pain relief or resolution of trigger points, and may induce a local myopathy.[39] It is also well-described that steroid medications may diminish the local healing response to the needling technique. The use of local anesthetic has been advocated with these injections due to the reduction in intensity and duration of post-injection soreness.[64] Fischer has also reported that local anesthetic will reduce muscle spasm, provide immediate pain relief, improve desensitization, and potentiation of the mechanical effects of the needling technique.[39]

After a complete discussion of the procedure with the patient, the areas of tenderness are palpated and the trigger points are identified. The skin is marked appropriately and prepped with betadine. A 25-gauge needle is then placed into the trigger point with injection of approximately 0.5 cc of 1% lidocaine. After infiltration of this discrete area of the trigger point, the needle is withdrawn into the subcutaneous tissue and then redirected in order to infiltrate the peripheral portions of the trigger point. Typically, a total of 2 to 3 cc can be injected into each trigger point. If a muscle twitch is elicited with injection of the initial 0.5 cc of 1% lidocaine, this volume alone may be sufficient for trigger point management. One to three trigger points are normally injected at each treatment episode. These injections may be repeated every one to two weeks depending upon the degree and duration of pain relief.

These injections are a component of a comprehensive management program. Medications such as acetaminophen and/or anti-inflammatory medication can be used along with physical therapy for modalities and manual therapy. It is essential that any underlying mechanical dysfunction be addressed in order to maximize response to the injection.

Potential risks with trigger point injection include bleeding, infection, intravascular injection of the local anesthetic, and allergic reaction to the local anesthetic. The contraindications of trigger-point injections include the use of anti-coagulant medication, evidence of dermatitis or local infection in the area of the injection, bleeding disorders, and known allergy to the local anesthetic.

8.5 Prolotherapy

Prolotherapy involves the injection of a sclerosing solution to strengthen the attachment of ligaments, tendons, fascial structures, and joint capsules.[89] The strengthening of incompetent tendons and ligaments is accomplished by creating an irritation by an osmotic gradient, thus stimulating proliferation of new cells. Hackett has reported that the newly developed cells strengthen incompetent tendon and ligament structures.[59]

The theoretical indication for prolotherapy is to correct the presence of hyperlaxity in the lumbar spine identified on physical exam. There is no objective consistent finding which positively predicts response to prolotherapy. This laxity is felt to be the cause of pain in the tendonoligamentous structures as well as in the deeper somatic structures such as the periosteum and periosteal attachments. The prolotherapy is felt to return the connective tissue length to its normal proportion and strength, thus allowing these structures to provide its normal skeletal support.[4]

As with any injection procedure, proper patient selection is essential. As mentioned previously, ligamentous laxity identified on examination is a specific indication for prolotherapy in the lumbar spine. Consideration of prolotherapy is made only after the patient has failed the more traditional forms of treatment, including activity modification, correction of postural deformities, medications, and physical therapy. In order to allow the natural healing cascade to proceed, injections are usually not initiated for eight weeks.[89] Empiric recommendations of prolotherapy injectionists is that if documented improvement is not identified after five or six treatment sessions, the technique should be adjusted or other diagnoses considered.

Injections of the lumbar spine can involve both acute and chronic back pain. The area of injection is determined by a focused physical examination in order to identify the abnormal ligaments which are felt to be the pain generators. Typically, multiple injection sites are identified. Common areas of injection include the iliolumbar ligament which is injected adjacent to the iliac crest. The posterior sacrum is an area with a large number of potential injection sites. Lumbar facet ligaments and intertransverse ligaments of the lumbar spine can also cause localized or referred pain and should be thoroughly evaluated as well. The sacroiliac joints and the sacroiliac ligaments can be injected to reduce SI joint pain and promote SI joint stability.

Reeves reports that the most common sclerosing agent injected includes 4 cc of 50% dextrose, 2 cc of 2% xylocaine and 6 cc of bacteriostatic water.[89]

This solution is based on the approach of George Hackett.[59] There is also a West Coast method that uses phenol or sodium morrhuate in place of dextrose.[29] The use of phenol or sodium morrhuate is rarely indicated due to potential risks and increased localized pain with injection.

Two randomized controlled trials have been published on prolotherapy.[69, 85] Ongley reported improved disability scores in the prolotherapy group at one, three, and six months from the end of treatment in chronic low back pain patients. Visual analog pain scores and pain diagrams also showed significant improvements with prolotherapy.[85] Klein identified improvement in both the treatment and control group, without either demonstrating a statistical advantage.[69] Collagen fiber diameter has been demonstrated to increase an average of 0.33 μm when injecting a proliferant solution of 15% dextrose, 1.25% phenol, and 12.5% glycerin weekly for six weeks.[68] Hackett and Coplans have reported an 80% or greater reduction of chronic back pain using prolotherapy.[25, 59] Statistically, a significant reduction in collateral and cruciate ligament instability of the knee has also been demonstrated with prolotherapy at two-week intervals on four occasions.[84]

Complication is rare when these injections are provided by an experienced clinician. The injection may increase pain for up to one week following the injection. As expected, the use of phenol can dramatically increase the amount of pain, both during and after the procedure. With lumbar spine injections, there have been reports of neurologic impairment from spinal cord irritation due to subdural injection.[65]

8.6   Intradiscal Corticosteroid Injections

The use of intradiscal steroid injections for management of lumbar pain was first reported by Feffer in 1956.[38] Sixty-seven percent of patients receiving the intradiscal injection of 50 mg of hydrocortisone reported rapid remission of symptoms in 24 hours. Only four of these patients had recurrent of symptoms at a maximum follow-up period of eight months.

A prospective, randomized, double-blind study completed by Simmons reported no statistically significant benefit with the use of intradiscal steroids.[94] Graham published a double-blind study comparing chemonucleolysis and intradiscal administration of hydrocortisone in the treatment of backache and sciatica.[50] In the hydrocortisone group, 20 patients received an intradiscal hydrocortisone injection (dosage of injection not reported). Fifty percent of the hydrocortisone group had "fair to good" response to the injection. Duration of pain relief is not reported. Wilkinson completed a study on 42 intradiscal injections performed on 29 patients with lumbar disc disease. All of the patients included had significant pain for at least six months and had failed aggressive medical management. In the group considered to have predominantly discogenic pain, 54% received good results lasting more than three months. Forty percent of patients with primarily radicular pain received good results lasting greater than three months. The only complications encountered in this series was an occasional spinal headache and reported minor menstrual irregularities in young female patients.[108] Kato has reported a reduction in pain, a diminution in the size of the herniated disc and decrease of signal intensity of the disc following intradiscal injection of 40 mg of methylprednisolone.[6] The conclusion of this study was that discography with intradiscal steroid injection produced a progressive degeneration of the intervertebral disc. Animal studies have confirmed that methylprednisolone acetate and polyethylene glycol do, in fact, cause degeneration and primary calcification of the disc.[3]

By selecting patients who have MRI-documented annular tear with high signal intensity, recent studies have shown that 33% of patients are reported subjectively as markedly improved greater than six months after the injection. Thirty percent of the patients reported improvement although it was for less than six months. An additional 35% did not report any change with the injection.[86]

The technique for diagnostic discography has been outlined in the previous chapter. The identical technique is used for intradiscal steroid injections. Steroid doses in available studies range from 40–80 mg. The only additional complications from this procedure would be the potential systemic side effects of the corticosteroids. There are no available studies documenting specific patient selection, number of injections indicated, or long-term outcomes.

8.7 Sacroiliac Joint Injections

In the previous chapter, Dr. Woodward has thoroughly discussed patient selection and the procedure for SI joint injections. Slipman et al. reported recently that the positive predictive value of physical exam findings, including SI joint maneuvers to determine the presence of SI joint dysfunction, is approximately 60%.[36, 81, 97] Therefore, when SI joint injections are completed, they are typically being done for both diagnostic and therapeutic purposes. This injection is usually considered in cases that have failed initial attempts of conservative management. Once proper needle placement is confirmed in the SI joint following contrast injection, the joint is then injected with 0.75 cc of long-acting corticosteroid, such as Celestone and 0.75 cc of bupivacaine or xylocaine. Volumes with this injection remain small due to the limited joint capacity reported to average 1.6 cc.[43] Repeat injections are determined by subjective response, with a limitation to maximum of three times per year.[8]

The effectiveness of SI joint injections in treating SI joint dysfunction is based primarily upon empirical evidence, considering that there are no well-controlled studies currently available.[37] The results with SI joint injections do appear to be favorable when used to augment other forms of conservative management. In a small double-blind study of 10 patients (13 joints), intra-articular injection for sacroiliitis provided a good result of 86% at one month, 62% at three months, and 58% at six months.[82] Bollow has reported a statistically significant reduction in subjective complaints for up to 15 months after SI injection.[14]

8.8 Lumbar Sympathetic Blocks

Lumbar spine pathology is rarely a cause of sympathetically mediated pain syndromes. However, sympathetically mediated pain has been reported in association with lumbar radiculopathy[9] and also following lumbosacral spine surgery.[111] The use of lumbar sympathetic injections in these conditions can be helpful from both a diagnostic and therapeutic standpoint. A positive response to the injection is determined by subjective reports of pain diminution, along with objective observation of improvement of lower limb temperature, skin color, and tolerance to passive range of motion. Additional injections are recommended if therapeutic benefit is documented. Ideally, sequential prolongation of pain relief between injections is documented which further supports the use of repeated injections. Lumbar sympathetic injections have the potential of relieving discogenic pain by blocking the greater rami communicans portion to the sinuvertebral nerve and direct branches from the greater rami to the disc.

8.9 Summary

Therapeutic injections are a component of a comprehensive management program. By reducing pain and inflammation, these injections allow the patient to participate actively in their treatment, minimizing pain inhibition. The effectiveness of these injections is compromised when used in isolation, and therefore must be used in conjunction with appropriate rehabilitative measures. When performing these injections, fluoroscopy is used to reduce the risk of complication and ensure proper needle placement. With current research strategies, available techniques will certainly improve, and as a result, patient outcomes should continue to improve as well.

8.10 References

1. Andrade, S. A. Side effects of epidurally administered celestone, *Int. Spinal Injection Soc. Publ.* 1(5) 1993.
2. Andrade S. A. Steroid side effects of epidurally administered celestone, *Int. Spinal Injection Soc. Newsl.* 1(5) 1993.
3. Aoki, M., Kato, F. et al. Histologic changes in the intravertebral disc after intradiscal injections of methylprednisolone acetate in rabbits. *Spine,* 22(2):127–132, 1997.
4. Banks, A. R. A rationale for prolotherapy. *J. Orthop. Med. (U.K.)* 13:54–59, 1991.
5. Beliveau, P. A comparison between epidural anesthesia with and without corticosteroid in the treatment of sciatica, *Rheum. Phys. Med.,* 11(40) 1971.

6. Bennett, R. The fibrositis-fibromyalgia syndrome, in Schumacher, R. ed. *Primer on the Rheumatic Disease*. Atlanta: Arthritis Foundation, 227–230, 1988.

7. Benzon, H. T. Epidural steroid injections for low back pain and lumbosacral radiculopathy, *Pain*, 24(277) 1986.

8. Bernard, T. N. and Cassidy, J. D. The sacroiliac joint syndrome: Pathophysiology diagnosis and management, in: Frymoyer, J. W., ed. *The Adult Spine: Principles and Practice*. New York: Raven Press, 2107–30, 1991.

9. Bernini, P. M. and Simeone, F. A. Reflex sympathetic dystrophy associated with low lumbar disc herniation. *Spine* 6(2):180–184, 1981.

10. Blanchard, J., Ramamurthy, S., Walsh, N. et al. Intravenous regional sympatholysis. A double blind comparison of guanethidine, reserpine and normal saline. *J. Pain Symp. Manage.* 5:357–361, 1990.

11. Bogduk, N. International Spinal Injection Society Guidelines for the performance of spinal injection procedures, Part 1: Zygapophyseal joint (blocks), *Clin. J. Pain.* 13(4):285–302, 1997.

12. Bogduk, N., Christophidis, N., Cherry, D. et al. Epidural steroids in the management of back pain and sciatica of spinal origin, report of the working party on epidural use of steroids in the management of back pain. Canberra, Australia: National Health and Medical Research Council, 1993.

13. Bogduk, N., Simons, D. G. *Neck Pain: Joint Pain or Trigger Point? Progress in Fibromyalgia and Myofascial Pain*, Voeroy, H., Merskey, H., ed. Elsevier Science Publishers, pp. 267–273, 1993.

14. Bollow, M. and Braun, J. et al. CT-guided intra-articular corticosteroid injection into the sacroiliac joints in patients with spondyloarthropathy: Indication and follow-up with contrast enhanced MRI. *J. of Comput.-Assisted Tomography* 20(4):512–521.

15. Boudin, G., Barbizet, J., and Guihard, J. L'hydrocortisone, intrarachniclienne ses applications cliniques en particular daus le traitement de la meningite tuberculouse, *Bull. Soc. Med. Hop. (Paris)*, 21, 817, 1955.

16. Bridenbaugh, P. O. Patient management for neural blockade: Selection management, premedication, and supplementation, in *Neural Blockade in Clinical Anesthesia and Management of Pain*. Philadelphia: J.B. Lippincott, 191–212, 1988.

17. Brower, A. C. Disorders of the sacroiliac joint. *Surg. Rounds Orthop.* 13:47–54, 1989.

18. Brown, F. W. Management of discogenic pain using epidural and intrathecal steroids, *Clin. Orthop.*, 129, 72, 1977.

19. Burn, J. M. and Langdon, L. Duration of action of epidural methylprednisolone, *Am. J. Phys. Med.*, 53, 29, 1974.

20. Byrn, C., Olsson, I., Falkheden, L. et al. Subcutaneous sterile water injections for chronic neck and shoulder pain following whiplash injuries. *Lancet* 341:449–452, 1993.

21. Carette, S., Leclaire, R., Marcoux, S. et al. Epidural corticosteroid injections for sciatica due to herniated nucleus pulposus. *N. Engl. J. Med.* 1997; 336 (23): 1634–40.

22. Carette, S., Marcoux, S., Truchon, R. et al. A controlled trial of corticosteroid injections into the facet joints for chronic low back pain. *N. Engl. J. Med.*, 325, 1002, 1991.

23. Carr, D. B. Epidural steroids for radiculalgia, *Journees de club anesthesie-douler*, 32, 289, 101.

24. Cohn, N. L., Huntington, C. T., Byrd, S. E. et al. Epidural morphine and methylprednisolone: New therapy for recurrent low back pain, *Spine*, 11, 960, 1986.

25. Coplans, C. W. The conservative treatment of low back pain. *The Conservative Treatment of Low Back Pain*. Philadelphia: J.B. Lippincott, 145–183, 1978.

26. Devor, N., Gourin-Littmann, R., and Raber, T. Corticosteroids suppress ectopic neural discharge originating in experimental neuromas, *Pain*, 22, 127, 1985.

27. Deyo, R. A. Conservative therapy for low back pain. *JAMA* 250:1057–1062, 1983.

28. Dilke, T. F., Burry, H. C., and Grahame, R. Extradural corticosteroid injection in the management of lumbar nerve-root compression, *BMJ*, 2, 635, 1973.

29. Dorman, T. A. and Ravin, T. H. *Diagnosis and Injection Techniques in Orthopedic Medicine*. Baltimore: Williams and Wilkins, 1991.

30. Dreyer, S. J. and Dreyfuss, P. H. Low back pain and the zygapophyseal (facet) joints, *Arch. Phys. Med. Rehabil.*, 77, 290, 1996.

31. Dreyer, S. J., Dreyfuss, P., and Cole, A. J. Zygapophyseal (facet) injections, intra-articular and medial branch block techniques, in: Injection techniques principle and practice, Weinstein, S. M. ed., *Phys. Med. Rehabil. Clinics, N.A.*, Philadelphia: W.B. Saunders Co., 715, 1995.

32. Dreyfuss, P. Epidural steroid injections: A procedure ideally performed with fluoroscopic control and contrast media, *Int. Spinal Injection Soc. Publ.*, vol. 3, 1998.

33. Dreyfuss, P. The sacroiliac joint: A review. *Int. Spinal Injection Soc.* 2:21–58, 1994.

34. Dreyfuss, P., Dreyer, S. J., and Herring, S. A. Lumbar zygapophyseal (facet) joint injections. *Spine* 20 (18): 2040–7, 1995.

35. Dreyfuss, P., Dreyer, S., Griffin, J., Hoffman, J., and Walsh, N. Positive sacroiliac screening tests in asymptomatic adults. *Spine* 19:1138–43, 1994.

36. Dreyfuss, P., Michaelsen, D. C., and Pauza, K. The value of medical history and physical examination in diagnosing sacroiliac joint pain. *Spine* 21:2594–602, 1996.

37. Falco, F. Lumbar injection procedures in the management of low back pain in Malanga, G. A. ed., *Low Back Pain, State of the Art Rev.* Philadelphia: Hanley & Belfus, Inc. 13(1):121–149.

38. Feffer, H. L. Treatment of low back pain and sciatic pain by the injection of hydrocortisone into degenerated intervertebral discs. *J. Bone Joint Surg.* 38(A): 585–592, 1956.

39. Fischer, A. A. Trigger point injection. *Physiatric Procedures in Clinical Practice.* Philadelphia: Hanley & Belfus. Inc. 28–35, 1995.

40. Flower, R. J. and Blackwell, G. J. Anti-inflammatory steroids induce biosynthesis of a phospholipase A2 inhibitor which prevents prostaglandin generation, *Nature*, 278, 456, 1979.

41. Fluijter, M. and Van Kleef, M. The RF lesion of the lumbar intervertebral disc, Naastricht, Netherlands, April 1994.

42. Fortin, J. D. The sacroiliac joint: A new perspective. *J. Back Musculoskel. Rehabil.* 3:31–43, 1993.

43. Fortin, J. D., Dwyer, A. P., West, S. et al. Sacroiliac joint: Pain referral maps upon applying a new injection/arthrography technique. Part I: Asymptomatic volunteers. *Spine* 19:1475–1482, 1994.

44. Fraser, R. D., Osti, O. L. and Vernon-Roberts, B. Discitis after discography. *J. Bone Joint Surg.* 69B:26–35, 1987.

45. Frost, F. A., Jessen, B. and Siggaard-Andersen, J. A controlled, double-blind comparison of mepivacaine injection versus saline injection for myofascial pain. *Lancet* 1:499–500, 1980.

46. Frymoyer, J. W., Pope, M. H., Costanza, M. C. et al. Epidemiologic studies of low back pain. *Spine* 5:419–423, 1980.

47. Gallagher, J. et al. Radiofrequency of facet joint denervation in the treatment of low back pain: A prospective LED, double-blind study to assess its efficacy. *Pain Clinic* 7:193–8, 1994.

48. Gamburd, R. S. The use of selective injections in the lumbar spine, Phys. Med. *Rehabil. Clin. North Am.,* 2, 79, 1986.

49. Garvey, T. A., Marks, M. R., and Wiesel, S. W. A prospective, randomized, double-blind evaluation of trigger-point injection therapy for low back pain. *Spine* 14:926–964, 1989.

50. Graham, C. E. Chemonucleolysis: A double-blind study comparing chemonucleolysis with intradiscal hydrocortisone in the treatment of backache and sciatica. *Clin. Orthop.* 117:179–192, 1976.

51. Gray, R. G. and Gottleib, N. L. Intra-articular corticosteroids: An updated assessment. *Clin. Orthop.* 177, 235, 1983.

52. Green, P. W., Burke, A. J., Weiss, C. A. et al. The role of epidural cortisone injection in the treatment of discogenic low back pain, *Clin. Orthop.* 153, 121, 1980.

53. Gunn, C. C., Milbrandt, W. E., Little, A. S., and Mason, K. E. Dry needling of muscle motor points for chronic low back pain: A randomized clinical trial with long-term follow-up. *Spine* 5(3):279–291, 1980.

54. Hackett, G. S. Joint stabilization through induced ligament sclerosis. *Ohio State Med. J.* 49:877–884, 1953.

55. Hackett, G. S. Shearing injury to the sacroiliac joint. *J. Int. Coll. Surg.* 22:631–642, 1954.

56. Hackett, G. S. *Ligament and Tendon Relaxation Treated by Prolotherapy,* 3rd ed. Springfield, IL: Charles C. Thomas, 1956.

57. Hackett, G. S. Prolotherapy in whiplash and low back pain. *Postgrad. Med.* 27:214–219, 1960.

58. Hackett, G. S. Prolotherapy for sciatica from weak pelvic ligaments and bone dystrophy. *Clin. Med.* 8:2301–2316, 1961.

59. Hackett, G. S., Hemwall, G. A., and Montgomery, G. A. *Ligament and Tendon Relaxation Treated by Prolotherapy,* 5th ed. Oak Park, IL: Gustav A. Hemwall, 1992.

60. Haddox, J. D. Lumbar and cervical epidural steroid therapy, *Anesth. Clinics. North Am.,* 10, 179, 1992.

61. Harley, C. Epidural corticosteroid infiltration: A follow-up study of 50 cases, *Ann. Phys. Med.,* 9, 22, 1967.

62. Hasselkorn, J. K., Ciol, M. A., Rapp, S. et al. Epidural steroid injections in the treatment of low back pain: a meta-analysis (abstract). Back Pain Outcome Assessment Team, Fourth Annual Advisory Committee Meeting, Seattle, 1994.

63. Helliwell, M., Robertson, J. C., and Ellis, R. M. Outpatient treatment of low back pain and sciatica by a single epidural corticosteroid injection, *Br. J. Clin. Pract.,* 39, 228, 1985.

64. Hong, C-Z. Lidocaine injection versus dry needling to myofascial trigger points: The importance of local twitch response: *Am. J. Phys. Med. Rehabil.* 73:256–263, 1994.

65. Hunt, W. E. and Baird, W. C. Complications following injections of sclerosing agent to precipitate fibro-osseous proliferation. *J. Neurosurg.* 18:461–465, 1961.

66. Kato, F., Mimatsu, K., Kawakami, N., Iwata, H., and Miura, T. Serial changes observed by magnetic resonance imaging in the intervertebral disc after chemonucleolysis: A consideration of the mechanism of chemonucleolysis. *Spine* 17:934–939, 1992.

67. Kepes, E. R. and Duncalf, D. Treatment of backache with spinal injections for local anesthetics, spinal and systemic steroids, a review, *Pain,* 22, 33, 1985.

68. Klein, R. G., Dorman, T. A., and Johnson, C. E. Proliferant injections for low back pain: Histologic changes of injected ligaments and objective measurements of lumbar spine mobility before and after treatment. *J. Neurol. Orthop. Med. Surg.* 10:141–144, 1989.

69. Klein, R. G., Eek, B. C., DeLong, B., and Mooney, V. A randomized double-blind trial of dextrose-glycerine-phenol injections for chronic low back pain. *J. Spinal Disord.* 6(1), 23–33, 1993.

70. Knight, C. L. and Burnell, J. C. Systemic side effects of extradural steroids, *Anesthesia,* 35, 593, 1980.

71. Kraener, J., Ludwig, J., Bickert, U. et al. Lumbar epidural perineural injection: A new technique, *Eur. Spine J.,* 6, 357, 1997.

72. Kraus, H. *Clinical Treatment of Back and Neck Pain.* New York: McGraw-Hill, 1970.

73. Kraus, H., Fischer, A. A. Diagnosis and treatment of myofascial pain. *Mount Sinai J. Med.* 58:235–239, 1991.

74. Kuslich, S. D., Ulstrom, C. L., and Michael, C. J. The tissue origin of low back pain and sciatica. *Orthop. Clin. North Am.* 22:181–187, 1991.

75. Lee, H. N., Weinstein, J. N., Miller, S. T. et al. The role of steroids and their effects on the phospholipase A2. An animal model of radiculopathy. *Spine,* 23, 1191, 1998.

76. Lilius, G., Laasonen, E. N., Myllynen, P. et al. Lumbar facet joint syndrome: A randomized clinical trial, *J. Bone Joint Surg.,* 71D, 681, 1989.

77. Liu, Y. K., Tipton, C. M., Mathes, R. D. et al. An in-situ study of the influence of a sclerosing solution in rabbit medial collateral ligaments and its junction strength. *Connect. Tissue Res.* 11:95–102, 1983.

78. Lofstrom, J. B. and Cousins, M. J. Sympathetic neural blockade of upper and lower extremity, in *Neural Blockade in Clinical Anesthesia and Management of Pain.* Philadelphia: J. B. Lippincott, 461–502, 1988.

79. Lynch, N. C. and Taylor, J. F. Facet joint injection for low back pain, *J. Bone Joint Surg.,* 68B, 138, 1986.

80. McCarron, R. F., Wimpee, N. M., Hudkins, P. G. et al. The inflammatory effect of nucleus pulposus: Possible element in the pathogenesis of low back pain, *Spine* 12, 760, 1987.

81. Maigne, J. Y., Aivaliklis, A., and Pfefer, F. Results of sacroiliac joint double block and value of sacroiliac pain provocation tests in 54 patients with low back pain. *Spine* 21:1889–1892, 1996.

82. Maugers, Y., Mathis, C. et al. Assessment of the efficacy of sacroiliac corticosteroid injections in spondyloarthropathies: A double-blind study. *Br. J. of Rheumatol.* 35:767–770, 1996.

83. Njoo, K. H. and Van der Does, E. The occurrence and inter-rater reliability of myofascial trigger points in the quadratus lumborum and gluteus medius: A

prospective study in nonspecific low back pain patients and controls in general practice. *Pain* 58:317–323, 1994.

84. Ongley, M. J., Dorman, T. A., Esk, B. C. et al. Ligamentous instability of the knees: A new approach to treatment. *Man. Med.* 3:152–154, 1988.

85. Ongley, M. J., Klein, R. G. et al. A new approach to the treatment of chronic low back pain. *Lancet*, 143–146, July 18, 1987.

86. Pollie, S. R. Current status of intradiscal procedures, corticosteroids, and radiofrequency, International Spinal Injection Society, Fifth Annual Meeting, October 4–5, 1997.

87. Raff, H., Nelson, D. K., Finding, J. W. et al. Acute and chronic suppression of ACTH and cortisol after epidural steroid administration in humans (Abstract), Program of the 73rd Annual Meeting of the Endocrine Society, Washington, DC, 1991.

88. Rapp, S. E., Hasselkorn, J. K., Elam, K. et al. Epidural steroid injection in the treatment of low back pain: A meta-analysis, *Anesthesiology*, 78, A923, 1994.

89. Reeves, K. D. Technique of prolotherapy. *Physiatric Procedures in Clinical Practice*. Philadelphia: Hanley & Belfus, Inc. 57–70, 1995.

90. Saal, J. S., Transon, R. C., Dobrow, R. et al. High levels of inflammatory phospholipase A2 activity in lumbar disc herniations, *Spine*, 15, 674, 1990.

91. Schwarzer, A. C., Wang, S., Bogduk, N. et al. Prevalence and clinical features of lumbar zygapophyseal joint pain: A study in an Australian population with chronic low back pain, *Ann. Rheum. Dis.*, 54, 100, 1995.

92. Shealy, C. Facet denervation in the management of back and sciatic pain, *Clin. Orthop.* 115, 157, 1976.

93. Shealy, C. Percutaneous radiofrequency denervation of spinal facets, *J. Neurosurg.* 43, 448, 1975.

94. Simmons, J. W., McMillin, J. N., Emery, S. F., and Kimmich, S. J. Intradiscal steroids. A prospective double-blind clinical trial. *Spine* 17(6 Suppl):5172–5, 1992.

95. Simons, D. G. Myofascial pain syndromes due to trigger points, in Goodgold, J. ed. *Rehabilitation Medicine*. St. Louis: Mosby, 686–723, 1988.

96. Simons, D. G. Muscular pain syndromes, in Friction, J. R., Awad, E. A. eds. *Advances in Pain Research and Therapy* New York: Raven Press 1–41, 1990.

97. Slipman, C. W., Sterenfelf, E. B., Chou, L. H. et al. The predictive value of provacative sacroiliac joint stress maneuvers in the diagnosis of sacroiliac joint syndrome, *Arch. of Phys. Med. and Rehab.*, 79, 288–292, 1998.

98. Slipman, C. W., Sterenfeld, E. B., Chou, L. H., Herzog, R., Vresilovic, E. J., and Abrams, S. The value of radionuclide imaging in the diagnosis of sacroiliac joint syndrome. *Spine* 19:2251–4, 1996.

99. Stambough, J. L., Booth, R. E., and Rothman, R. H. Transient hypercorticism after epidural steroid injection: A case report. *J. Bone Joint Surg.*, aq, 1115, 1984.

100. Takata, T., Inoue, S. Takahashi, K. et al. Swelling of the cauda equina in patients who have herniation of a lumbar disc: a possible pathogenesis of sciatica, *J. Bone Surg.* 70A, 361, 1988.

101. Travell, J. G. and Simons, D. G. *Myofascial Pain and Dysfunction: The Trigger Point Manual, Vol. 1.* Baltimore: Williams and Watkins, 1983.

102. Travell, J. G. and Simons, D. G. *Myofascial Pain and Dysfunction: The Trigger Point Manual, The Lower Extremities, Vol. 2.* Baltimore: Williams and Watkins, 1992.

103. Tuel, S. M., Meythaler, J. M., and Cross, L. L. Cushing's syndrome from epidural methylprednisolone, *Pain*, 40, 81, 1990.

104. Watts, R. W. and Silagy, C. A. A meta-analysis on the efficacy of epidural corticosteroids in the treatment of sciatica, *Anesth. Intensive Care*, 23, 564, 1995.

105. Weinstein, J. Mechanisms of spinal pain: The dorsal root ganglion and its role as a mediator of low back pain, *Spine*, 11, 999, 1986.

106. White, A. H. Injection techniques for the diagnosis and treatment of low back pain, *Orthop. Clin. North. Am.*, 14, 553, 1983.

107. White, A. H., Durby, R., and Wayne, G. Epidural injections for the diagnosis in the treatment of low back pain, *Spine*, 5, 78, 1980.

108. Wilkinson, H. A. and Schuman, N. Intradiscal corticosteroids in the treatment of lumbar and cervical disc problems. *Spine* 5:385–389, 1980.

109. Windsor, R. E. and Dreyer, S. J. Facet joint nerve ablation, in Lennard, T. A. ed. *Psychiatric Procedures in Clinical Practice*, Philadelphia: Hanley & Belfus Inc., 239, 1995.

110. Windsor, R. E., Falco, J. E., and Furman, M. B. Therapeutic lumbar disc procedures, in Injection techniques principles and practice, Weinstein, S. N. ed. *Phys. Med. Rehabil. Clinics, North Am.*, Philadelphia: W. B. Saunders, 771, 1995.

111. Windsor, R. E., Lester, J. P., and Dreyer, S. J. Cervical, thoracic, and lumbar sympathetic blockade, in *Physiatric Procedures in Clinical Practice*, Lennard, T. ed. Philadelphia: Hanley & Belfus Inc., 1995.

112. Winnie, A. P., Hartmen, J. T., Meyers, H. L. et al. Pain clinic II. Intradural and extradural corticosteroids for sciatica, *Anesth. Analg.* 51, 990, 1972.

113. Woodward, J. L., Herring, S. A., Windsor, R. E. et al. Epidural procedures in spine pain management, in *Physiatric procedures in clinical practice*, Lennard, T.A. ed. Philadelphia: Hanley & Belfus Inc., 260, 1995.

114. Woodward, J. L. and Weinstein, S. M. Epidural injections for the diagnosis and management of axial and radicular pain syndromes, in *Injection Techniques: Principles and Practice*, Weinstein, S., ed. *Phys. Med. Rehabil. Clinics, North Am.*, Philadelphia: W. B. Saunders, 691, 1995.

115. Zucherman, J., Dwyer, J., Hsu, K. et al. *Sympathetically Mediated Pain Disorders of the Lumbar Spine*. Boston: International Society for the Study of the Lumbar Spine, 4, 1990.

chapter nine

Manual Medicine

James W. Atchison, D.O.

9.1   Overview

Manual medicine is the general term that encompasses a wide variety of techniques involving practitioners using their hands as therapeutic tools to promote musculoskeletal changes in patients.[1] The term "manipulation" is most often used to describe the high-velocity or thrusting type of manual medicine that is performed by a variety of clinical practitioners including allopathic physicians, osteopathic physicians, chiropractors, and physical therapists. There are many other types of manipulation including articulatory, muscle energy, counterstrain, myofascial release, and craniosacral techniques. Soft tissue manipulation such as traditional stroking, compression, percussion, and friction techniques[2-5] performed by massage therapists may also be considered manual medicine. Acupressure,[6] Shiatsu,[6] Reflexology,[6] Rolfing,[7] and Bindegewebs massage[8] are more specialized forms of manual treatment which enjoy some degree of societal popularity. An estimated 12 million Americans[9] receive 90–120 million chiropractic manipulations per year[10] indicating the high demand for manual medicine[11, 12] from just this one area of practice. This number does not begin to account for all the other types of manual medicine practitioners or treatments performed. It is not known what percentage of manual medicine treatments are performed due to work-related injuries/problems or if there are specific types of work-related injuries that will respond to manual medicine techniques better than others.

Although manual medicine can be traced historically to Hippocrates (460–377 B.C.),[13, 14] the foundations of its use as practiced today originated with the nineteenth-century "bonesetters" of England (e.g., Richard Hutton, Wharton Hood, Sir Herbert Baker, and others[7, 13]), the creation of the principles of osteopathic medicine by Andrew Taylor Still, M.D., in 1874,[2] and the initiation of chiropractic techniques by Daniel David Palmer in 1895.[1, 13] Palmer felt that alterations (subluxations) of the spinal column led to abnormal neural function which causes disease. Therefore, treatment focused on removal of the subluxation by chiropractic manipulation (Table 9.1). Currently many chiropractors believe in a wider scope of practice utilizing physiotherapy, vitamins, electrotherapy, and diet to broaden their treatment regimens. Still's osteopathic philosophy stressed wellness and wholeness of the body and his use of manual medicine was based not only on restoration and maintenance of the normal structural-functional relationship within the musculoskeletal system, but also the neural-hormonal relationship with all other systems.[2, 13] This "holistic" approach to patients has been adopted by many medical specialties, and today many osteopathic and allopathic physicians incorporate various types of manipulation (Table 9.2) into treatment plans for musculoskeletal problems along with the other aspects of traditional medical care.

Both the osteopathic and chiropractic professions have utilized manual medicine extensively over the past century and have continued to try to establish it as an accepted part of medical treatment for musculoskeletal problems. This has been enhanced recently by the release of the Agency for Health Care Policy and Research (AHCPR) guidelines for the treatment of acute low back problems in the U.S.[15] and the recommendations from the U.K. Clinical Standards Advisory Group,[16] both of which support the use of manipulation during certain time frames of care. In addition, some large-scale reviews[17–22] of the literature performed by independent researchers have indicated effi-

Table 9.1 Examples of Chiropractic Procedure Types

1. Unloaded spinal motion
   * Continuous passive motion
     —Prone recumbent flexion/extension
     —Lateral recumbent side-bending
   * Manual flexion/distraction
     —Prone recumbent flexion
     —Prone recumbent flexion with side-bending
2. Manipulation procedures
   * Static high velocity, low amplitude thrusting (HVLA)
     —Prone recumbent thrusting
     —Prone recumbent cam-driven drop mechanisms
     —Lateral recumbent coupled postures
     —Upright seated rotational maneuvers
   * Dynamic motion assisted HVLA
     —Prone recumbent thrusting
     —Prone recumbent cam-driven drop mechanisms
     —Later recumbent coupled postures

From Triano, J. J., McGregor, M., and Skogsbergh, D. R. Use of chiropractic manipulation in lumbar rehabilitation, *J. of Rehabil. Res. and Dev.*, vol. 34, no. 4, 394–404, 1997. With permission.

Table 9.2 Examples of Osteopathic Manipulation Techniques

1. Thrusting
   • Mobilization with impulse or high velocity, low amplitude (HVLA)
2. Nonthrusting
   • Mobilization without impulse or articulatory
   • Muscle energy
   • Counterstrain
   • Functional indirect
   • Myofascial release
   • Soft tissue
   • Craniosacral

From Atchison, J. W., Stoll, S. T. and Gilliar, W. G. Manipulation, traction, and massage, in *Physical Medicine and Rehabilitation*, Braddom, R. L., ed. Philadelphia: W.B. Saunders, 428, 1995. With permission.

cacy in various patient subpopulations, primarily with low back pain, but also including neck pain[23, 24] and headaches.[21] The concepts, benefits, risks, and effectiveness of manual medicine have remained controversial within traditional medical training centers, but due to the high patient interest and recent guidelines, the number of allopathic physicians seeking continuing education or advanced training in this area is at an all-time high.

A difficult task in learning, utilizing, studying, and teaching manual medicine is to try to understand and effectively communicate exactly what is being manipulated. In the past, terms such as osteopathic lesion, subluxation, joint blockage, loss of joint play, and joint dysfunction were used to describe the problem areas.[25-27] The current term for these structural problems is somatic dysfunction, defined as "impaired or altered function of related components of the somatic (body framework) system; skeletal, arthrodial, and myofascial structures; and related vascular, lymphatic, and neural elements."[28] Somatic dysfunction on physical examination is manifested as Tenderness to palpation, structural Asymmetry, altered Range of motion, and Tissue texture changes (TART). However, even with standardized definitions and physical examination parameters, the ability to reliably use manual evaluation and treatment techniques is often determined by the "hand skills" and experience of the practitioner, both of which can often require years to obtain.

The goals of a practitioner utilizing manipulation or manual medicine are to reverse the somatic dysfunction by improving motion in restricted areas in order to "enhance maximal, pain-free movement in postural balance thereby optimizing function and to maintain optimal body mechanics."[25, 29, 30] The treatments attempt to both restore the mechanical function of a joint and normalize the altered reflex patterns of the surrounding tissues[25, 26, 31, 32] as evidenced by optimum range of motion, body symmetry, and tissue texture, and reduction in pain/tenderness. The current techniques to accomplish this were developed and published by recent pioneers such as

Bourdillon,[33] Dvorak,[29, 34] Greenman,[2] Grieve,[35, 36] Jones,[37] Maigne,[38, 39] Maitland,[40, 41] Mitchell,[42] Neuman,[25] and Ward.[43] These techniques are extremely varied, but most of the research that supports the use of manipulation has been done with the thrusting or articulatory techniques (see the Techniques section) for low back pain[44] and neck pain.[21] Few of these trials have focused solely on injured workers or evaluated return-to-work (RTW) or other occupational outcome parameters to determine efficacy.[45–47]

9.2   Specific Assessment Techniques and Contraindications

Assessment for somatic dysfunction starts with a detailed history and physical examination that emphasizes a comprehensive neuromusculoskeletal examination. Greenman[2] has outlined a "12-step" exam to screen for structural abnormalities (Table 9.3) that can be easily incorporated into a routine exam without increasing time dramatically. This screening exam will alert the practitioner to the regions of the body that will require a more comprehensive structural evaluation incorporating observation, palpation, and segmental motion testing to assess for tenderness, musculoskeletal asymmetry, altered range of motion, and tissue texture changes. Tissue texture changes are assessed by observation and palpation of the tissues, from the most superficial layers down to the bony prominences. Muscle, tendon, and fascia may show signs of vasodilatation, edema, flaccidity, contraction, contracture, and/or fibrosis through changes in skin temperature (hot or cold), moisture (sweating), bogginess, ropiness, thickening or firmness of muscles.[2, 25, 33] Range of

Table 9.3   12-Step Screening Examination

1. Gait analysis in multiple directions.
2. Observation of static posture and palpable assessment of paired anatomical landmarks.
3. Dynamic trunk sidebending.
4. Standing flexion test.
5. Stork test.
6. Seated flexion test.
7. Screening test of upper extremities.
8. Trunk rotation.
9. Trunk sidebending.
10. Head and neck mobility.
11. Respiration of thoracic cage.
12. Lower extremity screening.

From Greenman, P. E. *Principles of Manual Medicine*, second edition. Baltimore: Williams & Wilkins, 18, 1996. With permission.

motion assessment is performed grossly by observation and segmentally by palpation to determine multilevel versus single-level abnormalities and hypo-mobility versus hypermobility. This is done by assessing the relationship between the physiological motion (the end of normal, active range of motion) and anatomical motion (the end of passive motion which, if exceeded, leads to ligamentous damage, dislocation, or fracture) of an individual, while assessing for potential pathological (the end of range of motion is earlier than expected) barriers (Figure 9.1).[2, 25, 31, 33] The assessment for asymmetry should include observation of posture and positioning, palpation for tenderness, and testing for strength and muscle tone.

The structural evaluation should be used to determine the presence of somatic dysfunction to help determine what type of manipulation may be of benefit to the patient, and should be repeated following treatment to determine efficacy/benefit. Once somatic dysfunction is diagnosed, usually a variety of manual techniques may be used for treatment, but each of these

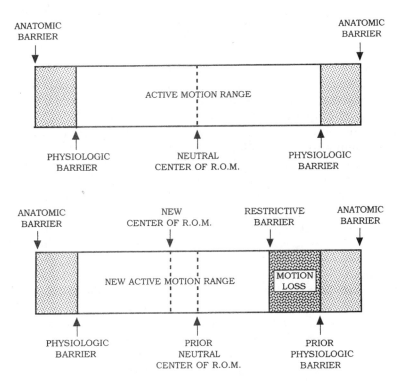

Figure 9.1 The barrier concept for normal joint motion (top) and with somatic dysfunction (bottom). All joints have an optimal range of motion with a physiological and an anatomical barrier at each end. A restrictive barrier causes motion loss and establishes a new center to the active range of motion. This shift in neutral positioning aids in the diagnosis of somatic dysfunction. From Kimberly, P.E., Formulating a prescription for osteopathic manipulative treatment. *J. Am. Osteopath. Assoc.* 79:508, 1980. With permission.

techniques has different indications and contraindications. Therefore, to decrease the risks and complications of manipulation, all information from the history and physical examination should be utilized to determine if there are any contraindications to a particular technique.[34]

Mobilization with impulse or thrusting manipulation (see the Techniques section) has the greatest number of absolute contraindications because of the sudden, rapid movement of the bones introduced by the practitioner.[14] These contraindications include malignancy, osteoporosis and all other metabolic bone diseases, fracture, aseptic necrosis, primary joint disease (rheumatoid arthritis, infectious arthritis), genetic disorders with hypermobility (Down's syndrome, Ehler-Danlos syndrome, Marfan's syndrome), aneurysm, congenital or acquired bleeding disorder, anticoagulant therapy, myelopathy, and/or cauda equina syndrome.[14, 48] Spondylolisthesis and acute herniated nucleus pulposus with radiculopathy may also be relative contraindications to thrusting techniques, especially for inexperienced practitioners.[14] Soft tissue, muscle energy, counterstrain, and myofascial release techniques (see the Techniques section) have few contraindications, because the motion during treatment is very slow and controlled with the patient providing much of the force involved.

Knowledge of the absolute and relative contraindications for each technique is essential before performing any type of manual treatment to limit adverse effects or catastrophic injuries. Severe, permanent sequela are estimated to occur in only one of every 1–1.5 million manipulations[9, 21, 49] and occur mostly with manipulation of the cervical spine by improper technique and/or inappropriate indications.[50–52] Reports of stroke,[21, 53–55] quadriplegia,[9] cauda equina syndrome,[9, 17] cardiac arrest,[56] and even death[21] are often the basis for most arguments against the use of manual medicine, but these events have been nearly eliminated in Switzerland by establishing rules for appropriate positioning and treatment.[57]

There have been reports of manual medicine causing less severe problems, such as progressive neurologic changes in a radicular pattern,[9] vertebral osteomyelitis,[58] compression fractures,[59] and worsening of herniated disks.[60, 61] Generally these syndromes have a highly variable course, and in most cases it is very difficult to determine whether the patient's condition worsened due to the manipulation or if the disease process continued through its natural course and the patient simply did not improve with the treatment. One of the most controversial areas concerning the use of manual medicine is in the presence of a known disk herniation.[44, 62] Nonthrusting techniques are typically preferred in these cases, but some studies on thrusting techniques in the lumbar spine have included patients with known radiculopathy who did not report any significant adverse outcomes.[63, 64] However, even the researchers in these studies have recommended the use of non-thrusting techniques[64–67] in the presence of known disk herniation, and sensory and motor status should be monitored correctly.

There are also a few general precautions to be followed for the safety and effectiveness of all manual medicine techniques. Positioning that includes any significant or prolonged neck extension should be avoided due to potential vertebral artery abnormalities and also the possibility of irritating arthritic facet joints or compressing the exiting cervical nerve roots in the lateral foramen. Prolonged or extreme neck rotation may also be dangerous in patients with carotid artery disease and should be limited because there is no reliable maneuver to test this prior to treatment. Extension maneuvers should be limited in the lumbar spine with patients who may possibly have central canal stenosis. In addition, all levels of the spine should be carefully positioned in persons with significant osteoporosis because rapid or prolonged flexion may lead to a compression fracture. With all techniques the patient must be kept relaxed and breathing freely to avoid excessive changes in blood pressure, as well as increased abdominal or spinal canal pressure.

There are potential side effects that can occur even when manual medicine treatment is appropriately indicated and correctly performed. These include a transient increase in discomfort[23, 24, 68, 69] and autonomic effects such as hypotension, flushing, altered menses, and increased perspiration. Because these effects can occur with appropriately administered treatments and because of the risk of catastrophic outcome, there is debate about whether specific informed consent in addition to the general consent to treat is necessary. This is an especially sensitive issue when treating injured workers who are often already involved in litigation, and there is currently no consensus among clinicians. At a minimum, it is recommended that discussion and documentation occur regarding the potential risks and benefits of this treatment as would be done to a similar degree with medications and other musculoskeletal treatments. Informed consent discussions may help a practitioner determine if the patient is truly a good candidate for manipulative treatment or whether more conservative, traditional medical treatment would be better tolerated.

9.3 Techniques

Manual medicine techniques are classified by the type of force utilized (intrinsic or extrinsic), the method of approaching the restriction or barrier (direct or indirect) (Figure 9.1), or the patient's contribution to the movement pattern (active or passive).[25, 30, 31] *Direct treatment methods*[2, 25, 30, 55] involve moving the patient toward the pathological barrier or in the direction of increasing resistance at the segmental level. Once the barrier has been engaged, force is applied to move through the pathological barrier toward the normal physiological or anatomical barrier (Figure 9.1). *Indirect treatment methods*[2, 25, 30, 31] involve moving the patient or segment in the direction of least resistance (away from the pathologic barrier) allowing the body's inherent and muscle energy forces to enhance mobility and create changes in the relationship between the position of the pathologic barrier and the normal physiologic barrier. *Extrinsic treatment forces*[30, 31, 33] are applied outside the patient's body and may be provided by gravity, straps, pads, or another person. The practitioner may use thrusting, springing, or guiding techniques to apply the force,[2] and patients are usually passive during these treatments. *Intrinsic treatment forces*[30, 31] occur within a patient's body and include muscle forces (active), respiratory forces (active), and inherent forces (passive) such as fluctuating body fluid pressures.[2]

Mobilization with impulse is commonly known as thrusting[70] or high-velocity, low-amplitude (HVLA) manipulation. These are the techniques most commonly associated with the term manipulation and often result in a "crack" or "pop" when a restricted joint is released.[71, 72] This is a direct treatment method that utilizes a very rapid, short duration, extrinsic force applied by a practitioner to a specific segment of a patient. The noise itself has no effect on treatment outcome; the benefit to the patient comes from the reintroduction of movement into the restricted or dysfunctional area.[70] HVLA techniques are most frequently performed by chiropractic and osteopathic physicians because they are the quickest mode of releasing a dysfunctional segment or region, but they also carry the highest degree of risk (see the Contraindications section).

When performing HVLA techniques, after ruling out absolute contraindications, the preparation of the patient is as important as the thrust itself[2, 25, 70, 73] (Figure 9.2). The more precise the positioning of the patient at the barrier in all three planes (flexion/extension, side bending, and rotation), the less thrusting force necessary for movement, and the force can be more specifically directed to the restricted segment. In general, high thrusting forces should be avoided to prevent possible soft tissue and/or joint injury, but the amount of thrust varies with the location of the treatment.[74] Treatment should always be provided in a pain-free direction,[25] so if a patient cannot be positioned without exacerbating the pain, a thrusting technique should not be performed. Pain in all planes may be an indication that the restriction is from a source other than somatic dysfunction (i.e., inflammatory/destructive process or nonphysiologic basis).[14, 75] Even when performed correctly, HVLA may not provide immediate relief of pain symptoms, but an improvement in the range of motion of the treated joint/segment should occur. This can only be determined by routinely repeating the structural evaluation after treatment.

Mobilization without impulse or articulatory techniques[2, 25] are passive, direct techniques that use a similar pattern of positioning and direction of force as HVLA. The most common form uses low velocity/low amplitude extrinsic forces to directly engage and then move away from the barrier.[40, 41, 76] By repeatedly "tapping" on the barrier, the technique is designed to improve the range of motion by gently moving the pathological barrier towards the physiological barrier[63] (Figure 9.1). A less common progressive or sustained loading technique may also be used.[77] Articulatory techniques require less extrinsic force to administer than the high velocity techniques and utilize some degree of intrinsic force in combination with the patient's ventilatory movement. In manual medicine literature these techniques are often just called "mobilization" or Maitland techniques,[65, 67, 78] can be performed at the time of diagnostic evaluation for range of motion in a given region, and can be easily combined with soft tissue or thrust techniques.[2]

The muscle energy (ME) techniques,[42, 79, 42] introduced by Mitchell,[80] involve a voluntary contraction of muscles (isometric, concentric, or eccentric) by the patient against resistance supplied by the practitioner. This is an active manual medicine treatment using predominantly intrinsic forces that can be applied to most muscle groups (spinal and peripheral) in the body as a combination of direct and indirect movements.[42] It is a relatively safe technique, with few contraindications because the patient controls the degree of force applied to the dysfunctional area. To perform a treatment, the patient is passively moved to the pathological barrier or restriction (may be in a single plane or all three planes), and then actively contracts his or her muscles in an attempt to move away from the barrier while the practitioner resists

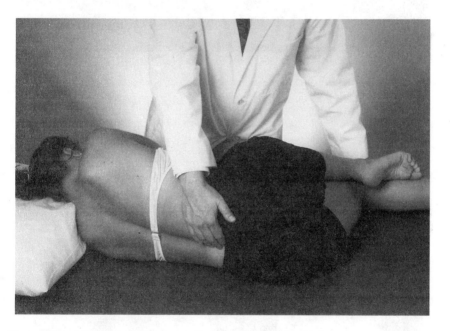

Figure 9.2a High-velocity, low-amplitude treatment for the lumbar spine with rotatory thrusting. *a.* The patient is flexed to the level of the barrier from below by using the legs and hips. The lower leg is re-extended and the top knee dropped to the table that adds right side-bending and left rotation below the level of dysfunction. *b.* From above, extension, right rotation, and left side-bending is incorporated by dropping the top shoulder posteriorly and pulling the inferior arm towards the practitioner. *c.* The practitioner thrusts by dropping his or her shoulders forcing the patient's shoulder toward the table and the hip toward himself or herself. From Atchison, J.W., Manipulation, in *The Nonsurgical Management of Acute Low Back Pain: Cutting Through the AHCPR Guidelines,* Gonzalez, E. G. and Materson, R. S., eds. New York: Demos Vermande, 187–197. With permission.

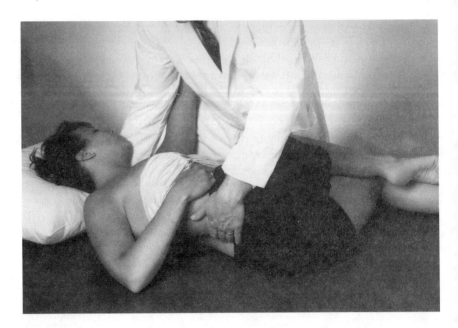

Figure 9.2b

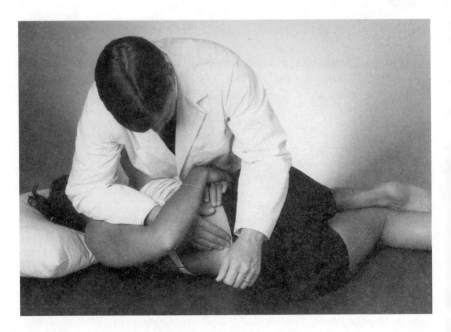

Figure 9.2c

(Figures 9.3 and 9.4). The patient tries to maintain a mild-to-moderate degree of sustained contraction for three to seven seconds. With instruction by the practitioner, the patient chooses the degree of active contraction, which should fire the muscle but not induce pain. The practitioner provides only static resistance and does not try to induce movement during the contraction. The more specific the positioning, the more localizing the contraction and the less force is needed. Following the contraction the patient completely relaxes the muscles, which usually takes one to two seconds, and the patient should not be moved during this time. Then the practitioner passively moves the patient to the new barrier. This step-by-step procedure is repeated three to five times, in an attempt to increase muscle length and advance motion past the pathological barrier towards the physiologic barrier following each contraction. Physical therapists refer to this technique as "contract-relax."[81] The goal is to increase the mobility of hypomobile segments, increase functional range of motion, allow the return of symmetrical motion to affected segments, strengthen weakened muscles, and lengthen contracted or hypertonic muscles.[2, 79, 82]

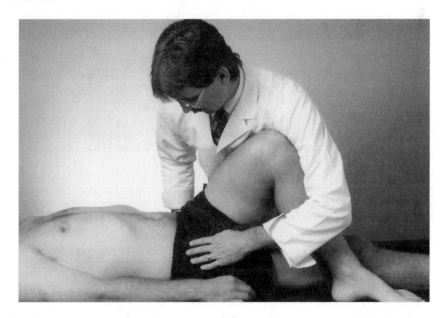

Figure 9.3   Thoraco-lumbar muscle energy treatment. When a structural examination reveals posterior rotation of the left transverse process or restriction of right rotation, this technique may be beneficial. The patient's left hip is flexed and adducted to the barrier without inducing pelvic motion. The patient actively abducts the hip against resistance by pushing into the practitioner's chest while the practitioner palpates the dysfunctional area with the right hand. From Atchison, J. W., Manipulation, in *The Nonsurgical Management of Acute Low Back Pain: Cutting Through the AHCPR Guidelines*, Gonzalez, E. G. and Materson, R. S. eds., New York Demos Vermande, 187–197. With permission.

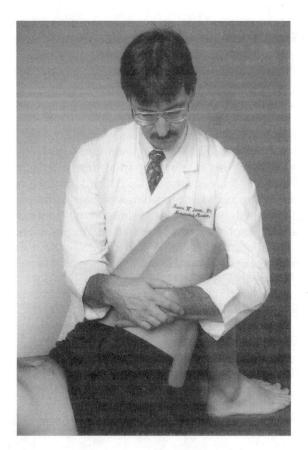

Figure 9.4a   Muscle energy treatment for the sacroiliac joint may include: *a*. Supine, resisted abduction (both hips); *b*. Supine, resisted adduction (both hips); *c*. Supine, resisted extension (left hip); and *d*. Supine, resisted flexion (right hip). These maneuvers are used in varying combinations depending on the patient's structural examination findings. From Atchison, J. W., Stoll, S. T. and Gilliar, W. G. Manipulation, traction, and massage, in *A Textbook of Physical Medicine and Rehabilitation*. R. L. Braddom, ed. Philadelphia: W.B. Saunders, 421–448, 1995. With permission.

Strain/counterstrain (CS) techniques attempt to passively place a spinal segment or other joint into its position of greatest comfort or ease. This is one of the indirect, "functional" techniques[2, 83] that was developed by Jones,[37] and utilizes extrinsic forces for positioning but intrinsic forces for release. The goal of the positioning treatment is to increase functional pain-free range of motion, relengthen contracted/hypertonic muscles, allow return of symmetrical segmental motion, and reduce pain through a reduction in inappropriate afferent proprioceptive neurologic activity.[26, 79, 84] The technique is very well tolerated by patients because it requires no active muscle movement or thrusting and relies on patient interaction to determine the position of maximum relief.[85]

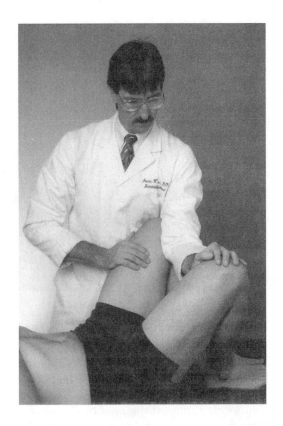

Figure 9.4b

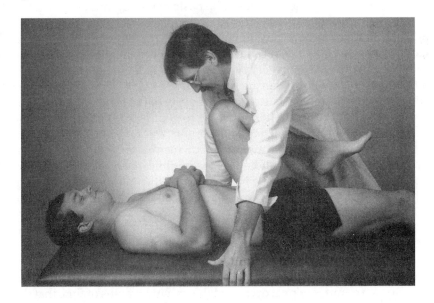

Figure 9.4c

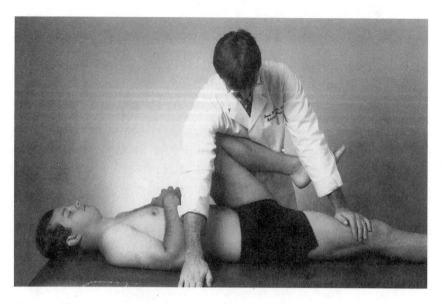

Figure 9.4d

Structural evaluation is required prior to using CS treatment to determine the areas of dysfunction and to identify "Jones/tender points."[37, 85, 86] The "tender points" are palpably tense; and tender areas located deep in the soft tissue and are not located only in the area of dysfunction. The practitioner uses one hand on the "tender point" as a "monitoring hand" while the other hand moves the patient through the basic planes of motion to localize the exact position that provides the greatest relief of pain to the "tender point" (Figure 9.5). Once the position of relief (ease) is determined, it should be maintained for 90 to 120 seconds, and then the patient is passively returned to the neutral position very slowly in order to let the muscle spindles reset themselves to their usual firing pattern in neutral.[26, 79] The patient must remain relaxed and should not assist by firing any of the involved muscles or the release will be impaired. After returning to neutral, the patient should be re-evaluated structurally as there may be other "tender points" that still require release or other forms of manual medicine that may be indicated. In general, the nearer the "tender point" to the midline, the more flexion or extension needed for relaxation. The more lateral to the midline, the more side bending (abduction/adduction) and/or internal/external rotation of the closest appendage will be needed.

There are few contraindications associated with counterstrain techniques, so the novice practitioner can safely perform them or incorporate them into a patient's home treatment program. There are limiting factors such as the time requirement to release multiple "tender points" (one and one-half to two minutes to treat each) and the varying lengths of time that the treatment may provide symptomatic relief (some may last only minutes). To

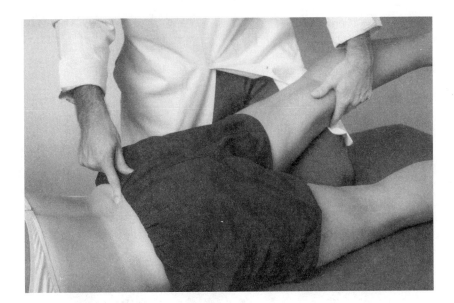

Figure 9.5a   Initial counterstrain position for treatment of: *a.* Right sacroiliac dysfunction. The position of "ease" is primarily an extension with slight addition of hip abduction or adduction. Note that the patient's thigh is resting on the practitioner's leg; and *b.* Anterior lumbar dysfunction with sacroiliac disorder. The position of ease is primarily trunk flexion (by flexing hips) with introduction of side-bending and rotation by the practitioner moving the patient's ankles toward or away from his body. Note that most of the weight of the legs is resting on the practitioner's leg. From Atchison, J. W., Manipulation for the treatment of occupational low back pain, in *Low Back Pain*, Malanga, G.A. ed. *Occup. Med. State of the Art Rev.* 13(1):185–197, 1998. With permission.

counteract these limitations, the CS techniques can either be taught to a family member to include with a home exercise program (HEP) or dosed appropriately by the practitioner to enhance the HEP. The dosing regimen should be considered carefully because some patients become "addicted" to this form of passive release and don't assume enough active responsibility for their own recovery.

The other *functional techniques*[2, 83] involve evaluation and treatment of the quality of motion of a joint or spinal segment instead of the absolute range of motion. The monitoring hand is placed over the dysfunctional segment to "listen" while motion is introduced into the area actively by the patient or passively by the practitioner. This "listening hand" is trying to determine which direction allows free and easy movement (ease) of the joint and which direction is difficult (bind). Motion is introduced in every direction in a sequential pattern while monitoring for ease in each direction. Functional techniques can be used in both acute and chronic problems because they are painless and depend on a release of soft tissue rather than a structural change.[2] The practitioner uses the listening hand

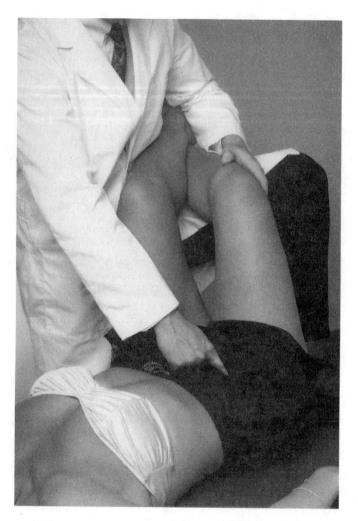

Figure 9.5b

to follow the pattern of ease which establishes improved motion throughout the joint/segment.

   Craniosacral therapy[2, 43, 87, 88] is a passive, indirect manual medicine technique using intrinsic force for diagnosis and treatment of the body by way of the primary respiratory mechanism. It was pioneered by Sutherland (1873–1954)[88] who perceived that the cranial bones undergo subtle cyclical motion about the cranial sutures at a rate of 8–12 Hz. The movement is felt most easily at the cranium and the sacrum, but is palpable everywhere in the body. He termed this inherent motion as the primary respiratory mechanism. Craniosacral therapy begins with assessing the amplitude, rate, symmetry, and quality of the primary respiratory mechanism, and then applying gentle pressure to the body in rhythm with the inherent motion. The patient is passively moved towards the position of optimal cranial and sacral mobility during the respiratory cycle.[87, 88] There is growing interest regarding the potential applicability and appropriateness of craniosacral therapy in patients following head trauma and with postconcussive syndrome,[89, 90] and chronic pain syndromes. However to date, despite some basic research on the movement of cranial sutures,[91-93] craniosacral therapy has more hypothetical than documented scientific support.

Soft tissue techniques are passive, indirect methods using extrinsic forces through lateral stretching, linear stretching, deep pressure, and/or traction that is directed at separating the origin and insertion of a muscle[2] (Figure 9.6). These techniques incorporate the principles of traditional massage techniques including effleurage or stroking, pétrissage or compression, tapotement or percussion, and friction, but may also include acupressure,[6] Travell's

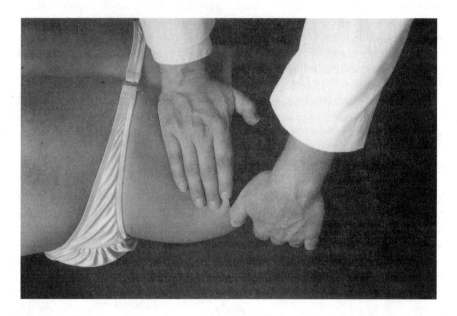

Figure 9.6 Soft tissue release by a combination of lateral stretch (cephalad hand) and rotary tractive fence (caudal hand). The base of the upper hand is placed just lateral to the spinous processes and makes contact with the border of the spinalis muscles. The hand is gently moved laterally (away from the practitioner's body) while maintaining contact with the medial border of the muscle. If the hand slips across the muscle, it must be repositioned. This technique may be performed alone or in combination with the fingers of the lower hand of the practitioner being hooked against the patient's ASIS and pulling backwards. The practitioner keeps the arm straight and leans back away from the patient at the shoulders. This provides a counter rotating tractive force to the upper hand. From Atchison, J. W., Stoll, S. T. and Gilliar, W. G. Manipulation, traction, and massage, in *A Textbook of Physical Medicine and Rehabilitation*. R. L. Braddom, ed. Philadelphia: W.B. Saunders, 421–448, 1995. With permission.

trigger point release,[94] diaphragmatic release,[2] mesenteric release,[2] or lymphatic drainage techniques.[2, 95, 96] Soft tissue techniques can be incorporated into generalized treatment programs for patients with musculoskeletal problems and are commonly used preceding other forms of manipulation, and should always be combined with an active treatment regimen.

Myofascial release[2, 7, 43] involves soft tissue treatment of the neuromuscular-somatic unit that combines "functional," muscle energy, and craniosacral principles. It uses intrinsic and extrinsic forces with direct or indirect methods to release somatic dysfunction or related imbalances affecting a discrete region, vertebral segmental level, or entire limb. Each of the techniques uses a combination of manual traction and twisting maneuvers to achieve tension on the soft tissues that will effect biomechanical and reflex changes.[2, 43] The direct form of myofascial treatment engages the restrictive barrier and pushes against it with a constant force until tissue release occurs, while the indirect technique guides the dysfunctional tissues along the path of least resistance until free movement is achieved. This is a dynamic treatment process that cannot be predetermined by the practitioner, but must be continually adjusted due to the response of the patient's tissues. Ward[43] and others have established general principles, but experience and expertise of palpatory skills are essential for a practitioner to obtain treatment success. This form of manual medicine is becoming widely used by physical therapists in both acute and chronic musculoskeletal pain syndromes, but is a passive approach to advancing range of motion and must be combined with an active approach to the patient.

9.4   Indications and Treatment Approach

Manual medicine techniques may be useful for the treatment of somatic dysfunction in any musculoskeletal region demonstrating a loss of functional range of motion, a change in tissue texture, or an asymmetry of structural or segmental motion testing. This can include spinal-related conditions such as cervical pain,[21, 39, 40, 97] thoracic pain,[38–40, 73, 98] rib strain,[2, 39] functional/mechanical low back pain,[20, 37, 38, 40, 73, 99–102] lumbar spinal stenosis,[103, 104] bulging intervertebral disc,[3, 39, 63, 105] facet syndrome,[37, 106] piriformis syndrome,[37] sciatica,[38, 63, 64, 66, 107] headaches,[21, 38, 39, 73, 87, 88, 108] and sacroiliac syndromes.[14, 37, 40, 73, 109] Manual medicine is only one component of a comprehensive treatment plan which may also include analgesic medications, modalities, activity modification, and an active exercise program involving both joint-specific or region-specific activities and aerobic reconditioning.

Treatment plans for all types of manual medicine must be developed on an individual basis in relation to the patient's structural diagnosis, the type and location of the somatic dysfunction, the type of manual medicine techniques being performed, and the patient's response to treatment. At each followup visit, the practitioner must re-evaluate these parameters to determine whether there is a need for continued manipulative treatment. Unfortunately, there are no well-controlled studies indicating the most efficacious frequency or duration of manipulative treatment, but the indiscriminate use of manual medicine for weeks or months without the proper indications is inappropriate. The RAND study[110, 111] made recommendations on the number of treatment visits a patient should receive based on classifying patients into clinical profiles of acute, subacute, and chronic pain. Some state and national practice guidelines have adopted these or similar regimens, but these are based on the opinions of expert panels only. It is recommended that if a patient is started on a course of manipulative treatment, there should be some demonstrable improvement within two weeks[44, 62] or the treatment should be discontinued and the diagnosis reassessed.

Therefore at each visit, the practitioner's goal is to determine by physical/structural examination whether or not there is a treatable dysfunction. If so, the treatment can be easily incorporated into the office visit immediately following the examination or the patient may be referred to a practitioner of manual medicine, either with a prescription for a specific technique or a request for an evaluation. The details of this referral relationship should be established prior to recognizing the needs of a specific patient so that each practitioner is clear on what is expected of the other and whom is managing the comprehensive treatment plan. Because manual medicine is only one part of the rehabilitation program for musculoskeletal pain, most often the referring physician should remain in charge of the program in order to prescribe analgesic medications, determine the need for other physical treatments or therapy, and determine current/changing physical capacities. Encouragement and reinforcement of the active HEP are essential to maintaining the increased range of motion and decreased pain that is acquired with manipulation. In fact, some forms of manual medicine (such as muscle energy and counterstrain) can be incorporated into a home treatment program along with the active exercise.[33, 112–114] This helps the patient actively participate in his or her treatment program and assume responsibility for recovery.

9.5 Patient Selection

When an injured worker goes for treatment during the first seven days following a discrete low back injury and the examination reveals localized pain and structural findings, manipulation and in particular HVLA may be considered for initial treatment if there are no specific contraindications. If there are contraindications to HVLA or if the pain complaints and physical examination findings are too diffuse, then nonthrusting techniques should be considered for initial manipulative treatment. Following a traumatic injury, such as a fall or being hit by an object, nonthrusting techniques may be better tolerated during the acute phase. However, with an acute muscle strain from a bending, twisting, or lifting maneuver, HVLA may be highly beneficial and tolerated. Whether the abnormal findings localize is an essential issue when determining if or what type of manipulative treatment may be most beneficial because an injured worker may manifest the negative psychosocial predictors of recovery even at the initial visit and will generally not respond to manual medicine any better than other forms of treatment.[115]

Localized rotational dysfunctions in the lumbar region, especially at L4–5 and L5–S1, respond well to the classic side-lying, rotatory thrusting or "lumbar roll position" (Figure 9.2). Some types of sacroiliac and pelvic dysfunctions are treated in the same position, while pelvic shears respond best to single, less distractive techniques in the supine position.[2]

The decision to include thrusting techniques in the treatment plan of an acutely injured worker should commit the practitioner to seeing the patient at least four to six times during the initial two weeks of treatment while the patient is also beginning an active exercise program. Thrusting manipulation is designed to enhance the effects of the active treatment program and is generally not felt to be effective on a weekly basis or a biweekly basis during the initial stages of treatment. The patient may be weaned to this type of regimen later in treatment; however, the goal would be to perform two to four HVLA treatments early in the hope that the patient will not need long-term treatment. The structural examination should be repeated at each visit to determine if the patient continues to require any further manipulation. The patient should continue the home exercise/treatment program while receiving all forms of manipulation and continue the program even after reaching a pain-free status. Often a patient will respond to treatment with fewer than four visits.

Muscle energy techniques are useful and effective in all regions of the body during the acute phase, especially in the thoracolumbar and the pelvic/sacral region. The lower thoracic/upper lumbar region responds well to the supine crossed knee-to-chest muscle energy technique (Figure 9.3) which can easily be combined with the thrusting techniques for the lower lumbar region. The pelvis/sacrum is perhaps the most difficult region of the body to treat and usually requires a series of muscle energy maneuvers which may be based on the screening/structural examination findings (Figure 9.4). Generally, the pelvis/sacrum cannot be treated alone, but must include treatment of the lumbar region and the lower limb. This is generally true for all of the transitional areas of the spine (cervical-thoracic, thoracic-lumbar, and lumbar-sacral). Acute hip problems would most likely respond to muscle energy treatment or myofascial release, counterstrain (Figure 9.5), and soft tissue techniques (Figure 9.6) combined with the muscle energy treatment, but are not very common in injured workers. Following treatment, if the structural re-evaluation indicates the patient benefited from a muscle energy or counterstrain technique, the patient may be instructed to include it in a HEP as a self-mobilization technique.

For a patient whose initial visit is two to six weeks after a specific work-related low back injury and whose pain has not localized, the nonthrusting techniques will often be better tolerated and more effective. In addition to the muscle energy techniques, myofascial release and counterstrain are particularly helpful because they involve an interaction with the patient regarding pain as the treatment is progressing. These are especially effective when a patient is extremely sensitive to palpatory maneuvers and could not tolerate more forceful movements. The pelvis/sacral/piriformis region also responds well (Figure 9.5). These gentle techniques often help a patient begin to improve his or her range of motion and reduce the pain enough to allow a more active program or a more aggressive manipulation program to be established. There can also be ongoing instruction to the patient for home use of the muscle energy and counterstrain techniques to be combined with the active exercise program. Because these treatments are passive in nature, a practitioner must be careful to objectively measure improvements following each treatment in order to determine if further treatments are indicated. If the patient is not making overall progress in his or her rehabilitation program, the manipulation should be discontinued because at times patients become dependent on manipulation just as they become dependent on medications.

When seeing new patients several weeks or months after their initial low back injury, the structural evaluation should be comprehensive because the patient is still symptomatic. Generally these patients have had multiple nonoperative treatment attempts and their pain complaints have become very widespread. Initiating manual medicine treatment at this stage should be carefully considered due to the often present psychosocial contributors to pain syndromes. If there are localized structural abnormalities and a previous manipulation treatment course has not been performed, manual medicine may still be of benefit.[22, 116] However, manipulation should not be attempted simply because it has not been tried. At this stage, manipulation should still be combined with an active exercise regimen, but generally a practitioner should consider a manipulative treatment course of 10 to 12 visits over six to eight weeks.

Treatment of persons with spontaneous onset of lumbar pain from an immobilization syndrome and not from an acute injury may respond very well to any of the manipulation techniques, but the symptoms will often recur if there is continued postural immobilization. Thrusting, articulatory, and muscle energy treatments are well-tolerated and potentially beneficial in this patient population, but the goal in treating these patients is to increase movement and encourage them to routinely perform their active exercise regimens. Aerobic activity should also be included in these treatment plans. Although passive in nature, myofascial release and counterstrain may help to improve the quality of movement in a specific region that allows patients to benefit more from their active treatment program. However, the manipulative treatment plan in this patient population should probably be limited to a burst of two to four visits over one to two weeks, which unfortunately may need to be performed three to four times a year.

9.6   Efficacy

The effectiveness and risks of manual medicine have been and continue to be intensely debated because, as with most other forms of conservative treatment of spinal and other musculoskeletal pain syndromes, good randomized, controlled studies to determine long-term benefits have not been conducted. The completed studies have been limited by the variability of the clinical problems (nonhomogeneous diagnostic groups), variety in the length of time with symptoms, the variety of manual medicine techniques utilized, the difficulty of blinding treatments, and the lack of widely accepted or validated outcome measures.[45, 66, 99–101, 117–121] There have been several recent reviews of manual medicine studies indicating effectiveness in certain subpopulations, especially in patients with low back pain for two to four weeks' duration.[19, 20, 122, 123] In addition to the usual questions regarding manipulation, there are even more specific questions to be answered about the efficacy of these treatments in the injured worker, and the low back region is the only area that has been evaluated.

Scheer[47, 124] reviewed treatments for low back pain that specifically evaluated return-to-work issues as the measurable outcome and only a single study was available. This study of automotive workers in Sweden by Berquist-Ullman[45] did show a positive benefit from thrusting manipulation for return-to-work patients, but the manipulation was combined with other nonoperative treatments. Scheer's review concluded that "randomized studies on spinal manipulation without co-intervention, utilizing work-related outcomes, are still needed to establish efficacy for acute LBP."[124]

Van der Weide's review[46] revealed three other papers[99, 125, 126] that correlated manipulation with specific vocational outcome parameters for acute low back pain. The most highly rated study[126] showed a positive effect for patients with pelvic dysfunction, and the paper concludes there is evidence of efficacy for spinal manipulation in chronic low back pain with pelvic joint dysfunction when compared to placebo. For other patients with short duration lumbar pain without radiating leg symptoms, there is moderate evidence that spinal manipulation is more effective than other types of nonoperative treatment in the short term. Two studies[126, 127] addressing vocational outcomes following manipulative treatment with chronic back pain were felt to be of low scientific quality, but Arkuszewski[128] did show a positive effect for improved rate of RTW compared to bed rest, analgesics, and massage only. Greenman[129] has demonstrated that attention and treatment to specific structural abnormalities of the pelvis and sacrum in persons with chronic low back pain may be of benefit in increasing the RTW rate even after years of disability. Patients without a discrete injury who develop diffuse soft tissue pain should be placed in a different category when being considered for manipulation as there has not been a clear benefit established in patients with a diagnosis of fibromyalgia.

There has also been recent interest in combining more aggressive nonoperative techniques for spine-related problems such as manipulation and epidural steroid injections,[130] manipulation and zygapophyseal joint injections,[106] manipulation and sacroiliac joint injections,[131, 132] and manipulation and lumbar sympathetic blocks.[133] Most of these reports include the use of active exercise programs following the initial interventions to assist with long-term improvement.

9.7 Summary

The use of manual medicine in patients with acute musculoskeletal injuries is becoming more routinely accepted and appreciated; however, the effectiveness of manual medicine with injured workers is limited by the same psychosocial variables that affect all other forms of musculoskeletal treatment. Therefore manual medicine should be performed only on injured workers who have somatic dysfunctions based on specific physical/structural examination abnormalities and limited evidence of pain behaviors or nonphysiologic sources of pain. For most musculoskeletal conditions, manipulation should be just one aspect of a comprehensive rehabilitation treatment plan and should be used only with an active exercise regimen. It takes years of hands-on experience to establish proficiency in certain manual techniques such as HVLA/thrusting, but the nonthrusting techniques may be easily and safely started on patients and many counterstrain and muscle energy techniques may be effectively and inexpensively incorporated into the patient's home treatment program.

Current studies support the use of manipulation to hasten the speed of recovery by decreasing pain, increasing range of motion, and improving function. Further studies are need in a population specific to injured workers which will establish the number of treatments necessary, beneficial, or cost-effective to returning the population to productive work activities.

9.8 References

1. Scientific Advisory Committee. International Federation of Manual Medicine, Workshop. Fischingen, Switzerland: 1983.
2. Greenman, P. E. *Principles of Manual Medicine.* 2nd ed. Baltimore: Williams & Wilkins, 1996.
3. Cyriax, J. and Russell, G. *Textbook of Orthopaedic Medicine, vol. 2: Treatment by Manipulation, Massage, and Injection.* 10 ed. London: Bailliere Tindall, 1980.
4. Hofkosh, J. M. Classical massage, in: Basmajian, J. V., ed., *Manipulation, Traction, and Massage,* 3rd ed. Baltimore: Williams & Wilkins; 263–9:1985.
5. Atchison, J. W., Stoll, S. T. and Gilliar, W. G. Manipulation, traction, and massage, in: Braddom, R. L., ed., *A Textbook of Physical Medicine and Rehabilitation,* 1st ed. Philadelphia: W.B. Saunders Co. 421–48:1995.
6. Tappan, F. *Healing Massage Techniques: Holistic, Classic, and Emerging Methods,* 2nd ed. Norwalk, CT: Appleton & Lange, 1988.
7. Cantu, R. L. and Grodin, A. J. *Myofascial Manipulation: Theory and Clinical Application.* Lewis, C. B., ed. Gaithersburg, Md: Aspen Publishers: 1992.
8. Dicke, E., Schliack, H. and Wolff, A. *Bindegewebs Massage,* 8th ed. Stuttgart: Thieme. 1975.
9. Powell, F. C., Hanigan, W. C. and Olivero, W. C. A risk/benefit analysis of spinal manipulation therapy for relief of lumbar or cervical pain. *Neurosurgery* 33:73–8, 1992.
10. Haldeman, S. Spinal manipulative therapy: A status report. *Clin. Orthop.* 179:62–70, 1983.

11. Eisenberg, D. M., Kessler, R. C., Foster, C., Norlock, F. E., Calkins, D. R., and Delbanco, T. L. Unconventional medicine in the United States: Prevalence, costs, and patterns of use. *N. Engl. J. Med.* 328:246–52, 1993.

12. Paramore, L. C. Use of alternative therapies: estimates from the 1994 Robert Wood Johnson Foundation National Access to Care Survey. *J. Pain Symptom Manage.* 13(2):83–9, 1997.

13. Harris, J. D. History and development of manipulation and mobilization. in: Basmajian, J. V., ed., *Manipulation, traction, and massage,* 3rd ed. Baltimore: Williams & Wilkins, 3–21, 1985.

14. Haldeman, S. Spinal manipulative therapy in the management of low back pain. In: Finneson, B. E., ed. *Low Back Pain,* 2nd ed. Philadelphia: J.B. Lippincott, 245–75, 1980.

15. Agency for Health Care Policy and Research. Acute low back problems in adults: assessment and treatment. *Clin. Pract. Guide Quick Ref. Guide Clin.* 14:1–25, 1994.

16. Clinical Standards Advisory Committee. Back pain: Report of a GSAG committee on back pain. HMSO, ed. London: 1994.

17. Shekelle, P. G., Adams, A. H., Chassin, M. R., Hurwitz, E. L. and Brook, R. H. Spinal manipulation for low-back pain [see comments]. *Ann. Intern. Med.* 117(7):590–8, 1992.

18. Assendelft, W. J., Koes, B. W., Knipschild, P. G., and Bouter, L. M. The relationship between methodological quality and conclusions in reviews of spinal manipulation [see comments]. *JAMA* 274(24):1942–8, 1995.

19. Anderson, R., Meeker, W. C., Wirick, B. E., Mootz, R. D., Kirk, D. H., and Adams, A. A. metanalysis of clinical trials of spinal manipulation [see comments]. *J. Manipulative Physiol. Ther.* 15(3):181–94, 1992.

20. Koes, B. W., Assendelft, W. J., van-der H. G., and Bouter, L. M. Spinal manipulation for low back pain. An updated systematic review of randomized clinical trials. *Spine* 21(24):2860–71, 1996.

21. Hurwitz, E. L., Aker, P. D., Adams, A. H., Meeker, W. C., and Shekelle, P. G. Manipulation and mobilization of the cervical spine. A systematic review of the literature. *Spine* 21(15):1746–59, 1996.

22. Anon. Acupuncture for low back pain: A systemic review. Manchester, U.K.: Third International Forum for Primary Care Research on Low Back Pain, 1998.

23. Gross, A. R., Aker, P. D., and Quartly, C. Manual therapy in the treatment of neck pain. *Rheum. Dis. Clin. N. Am.* 22(3):579–98, 1996.

24. Aker, P. D., Gross, A. R., Goldsmith, C. H., and Peloso, P. Conservative management of mechanical neck pain: systematic overview and meta-analysis [see comments]. *BMJ.* 313(7068):1291–6, 1996.

25. Neumann, H. D. *Introduction to Manual Medicine,* 3rd ed. Gilliar, W. G., ed. Berlin Heidelberg: Springer-Verlag, 1989.

26. Korr, I. M. Somatic dysfunction, osteopathic manipulative treatment, and the nervous system: A few facts, some theories, many questions. *J. Am. Osteopath. Assoc.* 86:109–14, 1986.

27. Korr, I. M. Proprioceptors and somatic dysfunction. *J. Am. Osteopath. Assoc.* 74:638–50, 1975.

28. International classification of diseases, 9th ed. *Clinical Modification,* 3rd ed. U.S. Department of Health and Human Services Publication No. (PHS) 89-1260, vol. 1:637; 1989.

29. Dvorak, J. and Dvorak, V. *Manual Medicine: Diagnostics,* 2nd ed. Gilliar, W. G., Greenman, P. E., eds. Stuttgart, New York: Thieme, 1990.
30. Greenman, P. E. Models and mechanisms of osteopathic manipulative medicine. *Osteopath. Med. News* 4:1–20, 1987.
31. Kimberly, P. E. Formulating a prescription for osteopathic manipulative treatment. *J. Am. Osteopath. Assoc.* 79:506–13, 1980.
32. Murphy, B. A., Dawson, N. J., and Slack, J. R. Sacroiliac joint manipulation decreases the H-reflex. *Electromyogr. Clin. Neurophysiol.* 35(2):87–94, 1995.
33. Bourdillon, J. F., Day, E. A., and Bookout, M. R. *Spinal Manipulation,* 5th ed. Oxford: Butterworth-Heinemann, 1992.
34. Dvorak, J., Dvorak, V., and Schneider, W. *Manual Medicine.* Berlin: Springer-Verlag, 1984.
35. Patriquin, D. A. Laterally transposed pelvis: A new and proper name for an old problem. *J. Am. Osteopath. Assoc.* 1992; 92:472–6.
36. Grieve, G. P. *Mobilization of the Spine: Notes on Examination, Assessment, and Clinical Method,* 4th ed. New York: Churchill Livingstone, 1984.
37. Jones, L. H. *Strain and Counterstrain,* 13th ed. Newark, OH: The American Academy of Osteopathy, 1992.
38. Maigne, R. *Orthopedic Medicine: A New Approach to Vertebral Manipulations.* Liberson, W. T., ed. Springfield, IL: Charles C. Thomas, 1972.
39. Maigne, R. Manipulation of the spine, in: Basmajian, J. V., ed. *Manipulation, Traction, and Massage,* 3rd ed. Baltimore: Williams & Wilkins; 71–134, 1985.
40. Maitland, G. D. *Vertebral Manipulation,* 5th ed. London: Butterworths, 1986.
41. Maitland, G. D. *Peripheral Manipulation,* 3rd ed. London: Butterworth-Heinemann, 1991.
42. Mitchell, F. L., Jr., Moran, P. S., and Pruzzo, N. A. *An Evaluation and Treatment Manual of Osteopathic Muscle Energy Procedures.* Valley Park, MO: Mitchell, Moran, and Pruzzo Associates, 1979.
43. Ward, R. C. Myofascial release concepts, in: Basmajian, J. V. and Nyberg, R., eds., *Rational Manual Therapies.* Baltimore: Williams & Wilkins, 223–41, 1993.
44. Atchison, J. W. Manipulation, in: Gonzalez, E. G. and Matheson, R. S., eds., *The Nonsurgical Management of Acute Low Back Pain.* New York: Demos Vermande; 187–98, 1997.
45. Bergquist-Ullman, M. and Larsson, U. Acute low back pain in industry. A controlled prospective study with special reference to therapy and confounding factors. *Acta. Orthop. Scand.* 170:1–117, 1977.
46. van-der Weide, W. E., Verbeek, J. H., and van Tulder, M. W. Vocational outcome of intervention for low back pain. *Scand. J. Work. Environ. Health* 23(3):165–78, 1997.
47. Scheer, S. J., Radack, K. L. and O'Brien, D. R., Jr. Randomized controlled trials in industrial low back pain relating to return to work, part 2, discogenic low back pain. *Arch. Phys. Med. Rehabil.* 77(11):1189–97, 1996.
48. Tobis, J. S. and Hoehler, F. *Musculoskeletal Manipulation: Evaluation of the Scientific Evidence.* Springfield, IL: Charles C. Thomas, 1986.
49. Dvorak J, and Orelli F. How dangerous is manipulation to the cervical spine: Case report and results of a survey. *Man. Med.* 2:1–4, 1985.
50. Curtis, P. and Bove, G. Family physicians, chiropractors, and back pain. *J. Fam. Pract.* 35:551–5, 1992.

51. Assendelft, W. J., Bouter, S. M., and Knipschild, P. G. Complications of spinal manipulation: A comprehensive review of the literature. *J. Fam. Pract.* 42(5):475–80, 1996.
52. Padua, L., Padua, R., LoMonaco, M., and Tonali, P. A. Radiculomedullary complications of cervical spinal manipulation. *Spinal. Cord.* 34(8):488–92, 1996.
53. Raskind, R. and North, C. M. Vertebral artery injuries following chiropractic cervical spine manipulation — case reports. *Angiol.* 41:445–52, 1990.
54. Sherman, D. G., Hart, R. G., and Easton, J. D. Abrupt change in head position and cerebral infarction. *Stroke* 12:2–6, 1981.
55. Krueger, B. R. and Okazaki, H. Vertebral-basilar distribution infarction following chiropractic cervical manipulation. *Mayo Clin. Proc.* 55:322–32, 1980.
56. Gorman, R. F. Cardiac arrest after cervical spine mobilization. *Med. J. Aust.* 2:169–70, 1978.
57. Inappropriate indications and contraindications for manual therapy. *Manual Med.* 6:85–8, 1991.
58. Lewis, M. and Grundy, D. Vertebral osteomyelitis following manipulation of spondylitic necks — a possible risk. *Paraplegia* 30:788–90, 1992.
59. Haldeman, S. and Rubinstein, S. M. Compression fractures in patients undergoing spinal manipulative therapy. *J. Manipulative Physiol. Ther.* 15:450–4, 1992.
60. Richard, J. Disk rupture with cauda equina syndrome after chiropractic adjustment. *N.Y. State J. Med.* 67:2496–8, 1967.
61. Hooper, J. Low back pain and manipulation: Paraparesis after treatment of low back pain by physical methods. *Med. J. Aust.* 1:549–51, 1973.
62. Triano, J. J., McGregor, M., and Skogsbergh, D. R. Use of chiropractic manipulation in lumbar rehabilitation. *J. Rehabil. Res. Dev.* 34(4):394–404, 1997.
63. Nwuga, V. C. B. Relative therapeutic efficacy of vertebral manipulation and conventional treatment in back pain management. *Am. J. Phys. Med. Rehabil.* 6:273–8, 1982.
64. Postacchini, F., Facchini, M., and Palieri, P. Efficacy of various forms of conservative treatment in low back pain. A comparative study. *Neuro-Orthopedics* 6(1):28–35, 1988.
65. Coxhead, C. E., Meade, T. W., Inskip, H., North, W. R. S., and Troup, J. D. G. Multicentre trial of physiotherapy in the management of sciatic symptoms. *Lancet* 1065–8, 1981.
66. MacDonald, R. S. and Bell, C. M. An open controlled assessment of osteopathic manipulation in nonspecific low back pain [published erratum appears in *Spine* 16(1):104, 1991]. *Spine* 15(5):364–70, 1990.
67. Edwards, B. C. Low back pain and pain resulting from lumbar spine conditions. *Aust. J. Physiother.* 15(3):104–10, 1969.
68. Haldeman, S. and Rubinstein, S. M. The precipitation or aggravation of musculoskeletal pain in patients receiving spinal manipulative therapy. *J. Manipulative Physiol. Ther.* 16:47–50, 1993.
69. Senstad, O., Leboeuf, Y. de C., and Borchgrevink, C. F. Side effects of chiropractic spinal manipulation: Types, frequency, discomfort, and course. *Scand. J. Prim. Health Care* 14(1):50–3, 1996.
70. Heilig, D. The thrust technique. *J. Am. Osteopath. Assoc.* 81:244–8, 1981.
71. Meal, G. M. and Scott, R. A. Analysis of the joint crack by simultaneous recording of sound and tension. *J. Manipulative Physiol. Ther.* 9:189–95, 1986.

72. Sandoz, R. The significance of the manipulative crack and of other articular noises. *Ann. Swiss Chiro. Assoc.* 4:47–68, 1969.

73. Fisk, J. W. *Medical Treatment of Neck and Back Pain.* Springfield, IL: Charles C. Thomas, 1987.

74. Herzog, W., Conway, P. J., Kawchuk, G. N., Zhang, Y., and Hasler, E. M. Forces exerted during spinal manipulative therapy. *Spine* 18:1206–12, 1993.

75. Waddell, G., McCulloch, J. A., Kummel, E., and Venner, R. M. Nonorganic physical signs in low back pain. *Spine* 5(2):117–25, 1980.

76. Nwuga, V. C. B. *Manipulation of the Spine.* Baltimore: Williams & Wilkins, 1976.

77. Nyberg, R. Manipulation: Definition, types, application, in: Basmajian, J. V., Nyberg, R., eds., *Rational Manual Therapies.* Baltimore: Williams & Wilkins, 21–17:1993.

78. Farrell, J. P. and Twomey, L. T. Acute low back pain. Comparison of two conservative treatment approaches. *Med. J. Aust.* 1(4):160–4, 1982.

79. Goodridge, J. P. Muscle energy technique: definition, explanation, methods of procedure. *J. Am. Osteopath. Assoc.* 81:249–54, 1981.

80. Mitchell, F. L., Sr. Structural pelvic function. *AAO Yearbook* 71–89, 1958.

81. Tanigawa, M. C. Comparison of the hold-relax procedure and passive mobilization on increasing muscle length. *Phys. Ther.* 52:725–35, 1972.

82. Hanten, W. P. and Chandler, S. D. Effects of myofascial release leg pull and sagittal plane isometric contract-relax techniques on passive straight-leg raise angle. *J. Orthop. Sports Phys. Ther.* 20(3):138–44, 1994.

83. Bowles, C. H. Functional technique: A modern perspective. *J. Am. Osteopath. Assoc.* 80:326–31, 1981.

84. Patterson, M. M. Louisa Burns Memorial Lecture 1980: The spinal cord — Active processor not passive transmitter. *J. Am. Osteopath. Assoc.* 80:210–5, 1980.

85. Brandt, B., Jr., and Jones, L. H. Some methods of applying counterstrain. *J. Am. Osteopath. Assoc.* 75:786–9, 1976.

86. Cislo, S., Ramirez, M. A., and Schwartz, H. R. Low back pain: Treatment of forward and backward sacral torsions using counterstrain. *J. Am. Osteopath. Assoc.* 91:255–9, 1991.

87. Upledger, J. E. and Vredevoogd, J. D. *Craniosacral Therapy.* Seattle: Eastland Press, 1983.

88. Sutherland Cranial Teaching Foundation of The Cranial Academy. *Osteopathy in the Cranial Field,* 3rd ed. Magoun, HI, ed. Kirksville, MO: The Journal Printing Company, 1976.

89. Greenman, P. E. and McPartland, J. M. Cranial findings and iatrogenesis from craniosacral manipulation in patients with traumatic brain syndrome. *J. Am. Osteopath. Assoc.* 95(3):182–8, 1995.

90. Greenman, P. E. *Craniosacral Manipulation in Persons with Traumatic Brain Injury.* East Lansing, MI: Kellogg Center, 1991.

91. Adams, T., Heisey, R. S., Smith, M. C., and Briner, B. J. Parietal bone mobility in the anesthetized cat. *J. Am. Osteopath. Assoc.* 92:599–622, 1992.

92. Norton, J. M. A tissue pressure model for palpatory perception of the cranial rhythmic impulse. *J. Am. Osteopath. Assoc.* 91:975–94, 1991.

93. Greenman, P. E. Roentgen findings in the craniosacral mechanism. *J. Am. Osteopath. Assoc.* 70(1):60–71, 1970.

94. Travell, J. and Simonsen, M. *Myofascial Pain and Dysfunction: The Trigger Point Manual.* Baltimore: Williams & Wilkins, 1983.

95. Zanolla, R., Monzeglio, C., Balzarini, A., and Martino, G. Evaluation of the results of three different methods of postmastectomy lymphedema treatment. *J. Surg. Onc.* 26:210–3, 1984.

96. Kurz, W., Litmanovitch, Y. I., Romanoff, H., Pfeifer, Y. and Sulman, F. G. Effect of manual lymphodrainage massage on blood components and urinary neurohormones in chronic lymphedema. *Angiol.* 32:119–27, 1981.

97. Beal, M. C., Vorro, J., and Johnston, W. L. Chronic cervical dysfunction: Correlation of myoelectric findings with clinical progress. *J. Am. Osteopath. Assoc.* 89:891–900, 1989.

98. DeFranca, G. G. and Levine, L. J. The T4 syndrome. *J. Manipulative Physiol. Ther.* 18(1):34–7, 1995.

99. Blomberg, S., Svardsudd, K., and Mildenberger, F. A controlled, multicentre trial of manual therapy in low back pain. Initial status, sick leave and pain score during follow-up. *Scand. J. Prim. Health Care* 10(3):170–8, 1992.

100. Meade, T. W., Dyer, S., Browne, W., Townsend, J., and Frank, A. O. Low back pain of mechanical origin: Randomized comparison of chiropractic and hospital outpatient treatment. *Br. Med. J.* 300:1431–7, 1990.

101. Hoehler, F. K., Tobis, J. S., and Buerger, A. A. Spinal manipulation for low back pain. *JAMA* 245:1835–8, 1981.

102. Assendelft, W. J., Koes, B. W., van der Heijden, G. J., and Bouter, L. M. The efficacy of chiropractic manipulation for back pain: Blinded review of relevant randomized clinical trials. *J. Manipulative Physiol. Ther.* 15(8):487–94, 1992.

103. Kirkaldy-Willis, W. H., Paine, K. W. E. and Candoix, J. Lumbar spine stenosis. *Clin. Orthop.* 99:30–50, 1974.

104. Atlas, S. J., Deyo, R. A., Keller, R. B., Chapin, A. M., Patrick, D. L., Long, J. M., and Singer, D. E. The Maine lumbar spine study, part III. One-year outcomes of surgical and nonsurgical management of lumbar spinal stenosis. *Spine* 21(15):1787–94, 1996.

105. Cyriax, J. Conservative treatment of lumbar disc lesions. *Physiotherapy* 50:300–3, 1964.

106. Dreyfuss, P., Michaelsen, M., and Horne, M. MUJA: Manipulation under joint anesthesia/analgesia: A treatment approach for recalcitrant low back pain of synovial joint origin. *J. Manipulative Physiol. Ther.* 18(8):537–46, 1995.

107. Atlas, S. J., Deyo, R. A., Keller, R. B., Chapin, A. M., Patrick, D. L., Long, J. M., and Singer, D. E. The Maine lumbar spine study, part II. One-year outcomes of surgical and nonsurgical management of sciatica. *Spine* 21(15):1777–86, 1996 Aug 1.

108. Nilsson, N. A randomized controlled trial of the effect of spinal manipulation in the treatment of cervicogenic headache. *J. Manipulative Physiol. Ther.* 18(7):435–40, 1995.

109. Vleeming, A., Mooney, V., Snijders, C., and Dorman, T. E. First interdisciplinary world congress on low back pain and its relation to the sacroillac joint, San Diego, 1992.

110. Shekelle, P. G., Adams, A. H., Chassin, M. R., Hurwitz, E. L., Park, R. E., and Phillips, R. B. *The Appropriateness of Spinal Manipulation for Low-Back Pain: Indications and Ratings by a Multidisciplinary Panel.* Santa Monica, CA: RAND Corp., 1991.

111. Shekelle, P. G., Adams, A. H., Chassin, M. R., Hurwitz, E. L., Park, R. E., and Phillips, R. B. *The Appropriateness of Spinal Manipulation for Low Back Pain:*

Indications and Ratings by an All-Chiropractic Expert Panel. Santa Monica, CA: RAND Corp., 1992.

112. Khalil, T. M., Asfour, S. S., Martinez, L. M., Waly, S. M., Rosomoff, R. S., and Rosomoff, H. L. Stretching in the rehabilitation of low-back pain patients. *Spine* 17:311–7, 1992.

113. Sweeney, T. Neck school: Cervicothoracic stabilization training. *Occup. Med. State of the Art Rev.* 7:43–54, 1992.

114. Erhard, R. E., Delitto, A., and Cibulka, M. T. Relative effectiveness of an extension program and a combined program of manipulation and flexion and extension exercises in patients with acute low back syndrome. *Phys. Ther.* 74(12):1093–100, 1994.

115. Gatchel, R. J., Polatin, P. B., and Mayer, T. G. The dominant role of psychosocial risk factors in the development of chronic low back pain disability. *Spine* 20:2702–9, 1995.

116. Wreje, U., Nordgren, B., and Aberg, H. Treatment of pelvic joint dysfunction in primary care — a controlled study. *Scand. J. Prim. Health Care* 10:310–5, 1992.

117. Sims-Williams, H., Jayson, M. I. V. and Young, S. M. S., Baddeley, H., and Collins, E. Controlled trial of mobilization and manipulation for low back pain: hospital patients. *Br. Med. J.* 2:1318–20, 1979.

118. Godfrey, C. M., Morgan, P. P., and Schatzker, J. A randomized trial of manipulation for low back pain in a medical setting. *Spine* 9:301–4, 1984.

119. Hidalgo, J. A., Genaidy, A. M., Huston, R., and Arantes, J. Occupational biomechanics of the neck: A review and recommendations. *J. Hum. Ergol. Tokyo* 21(2):165–81, 1992.

120. Fisk, J. W. A controlled trial of manipulation in a selected group of patients with low-back pain favoring one side. *N. Z. Med. J.* 10:288–91, 1979.

121. Blomberg, S., Hallin, G., Grann, K., Berg, E., and Sennerby, U. Manual therapy with steroid injections — a new approach to treatment of low back pain. *Spine* 19(5):569–77, 1994.

122. Koes, B. W., Bowler, L. M., and Kripschild, P. G. Spinal manipulation and mobilization for back and neck pain: An indexed review. *Br. Med. J.* 303:1298–303, 1991.

123. Shekelle, P. G. Spine update spinal manipulation. *Spine* 19:858–61, 1994.

124. Scheer, S. J., Radack, K. L., and O'Brien, D. R., Jr. Randomized controlled trials in industrial low back pain relating to return to work, part 1. Acute interventions. *Arch. Phys. Med. Rehabil.* 76(10):966–73, 1995.

125. Rasmussen, G. G. Manipulation in treatment of low back pain (a randomized clinical trial). *Man. Med.* 1:8–10, 1979.

126. Wreje, U., Nordgren, B. and Aberg H. Treatment of pelvic joint dysfunction in primary care — a controlled study [published erratum appears in *Scand. J. Prim. Health Care* 11(1):25, 1993.]. *Scand. J. Prim. Health Care* 10(4):310–5, 1992.

127. Gibson, T., Grahame, R., Harkness, J., Woo, P., Blagrave, P., and Hills, R. Controlled comparison of short-wave diathermy treatment with osteopathic treatment in non-specific low back pain. *Lancet* 1(8440):1258–61, 1985.

128. Arkuszewski, Z. The efficacy of manual treatment in low back pain: a clinical trial. *Man. Med.* 268–71, 1986.

129. Greenman, P. E. Kraft, GHSDFMEA, ed. Syndromes of the lumbar spine, pelvis, and sacrum. *Physical Medicine and Rehabilitation Clinics of North America: Manual Medicine.* Philadelphia: W. B. Saunders, 7(4):773, 1996.

130. Nelson, L., Aspergen, D., and Bova, C. The use of epidural steroid injection and manipulation on patients with chronic low back pain. *J. Manipulative Physiol. Ther.* 20(4):263–6, 1997.
131. Ongley, M. J., Klein, R. G., Dorman, T. A., Eek, B. C., and Hubert, L. J. A new approach to the treatment of chronic low back pain. *Lancet* 2(8551):143–6, 1987.
132. Dreyfuss, P., Cole, A. J., and Pauza, K. Sacroiliac joint injection techniques. in: Weinstein S. M. ed., *Injection Techniques: Principles and Practice.* Philadelphia: W. B. Saunders, p 785–813, 1995.
133. Braunstein, E. M., Cardinal, E., Buckwalter, K. A., and Capello, W. Bupivicaine arthrography of the postarthroplasty hip. *Skeletal. Radiol.* 24(7):519–21, 1995.

chapter ten

The Use of Physical Modalities for Occupational Low Back Pain

Myron M. LaBan, M.D.
Prathima Reddy, M.D.
Boris Terebuh, M.D.

10.1 Overview

Physical agent modalities are frequently utilized in the treatment of low back pain. Some treatment regimens rely wholly or significantly upon their use while other regimens rely upon them as a component of a multifaceted treatment strategy. This chapter will outline the commonly employed physical agent modalities for the treatment of low back pain.

10.2 Therapeutic Heat

Historically, heat in the form of hot water, vapor baths, heated sand, stones, oil, grain, salt, or other solids and liquids were the most frequent sources of therapeutic heat. Of the heating agents, hot water was the favored modality. Hippocrates advocated the application of hot water bags for sciatica. Hot sand baths were popular in the mid- to late 1800s and were widely available in both Europe and Russia. In 1893, Salaghi designed a heating pad which in 1895 was improved by Cerutti. In 1898, Von Leyden and Goldscheider described the benefits of warm water exercises, and Preiss invented the first electric-driven whirlpool bath which was used widely in France during World War I by military physicians. In the 1800s, the discovery of electricity rapidly gave impetus to therapeutic electrical heating. In 1875, Kellogg

0-8493-0089-4/00/$0.00+$.50
© 2000 by CRC Press LLC

developed a rectangular heating cabinet which employed 40-watt lamps and a reflector.[2] In 1928, Dr. Walter Blount devised the Hubbard tank which was initially used for underwater exercises and later as a source for therapeutic heat.

10.2.1 Heat Transfer

The transfer of heat to the lumbar region can occur by several mechanisms including conduction, convection, conversion, and radiation. Conduction transfers heat between two entities in direct contact. Convection utilizes a moving medium such as air or water to transfer heat. Conversion occurs when energy in the form of sound or electromagnetic energy is converted into thermal energy. Radiation takes place when thermal energy is emitted from one entity to another. The many mechanisms of heat penetrate the human body to varying depths. The modalities have therefore been categorized as superficial or deep heating modalities.

10.2.2 Superficial Heat

Hot packs typically contain a heat-retaining substance which is enclosed in a canvas bag. The hot packs are stored in heated water tanks and applied indirectly to the skin on a layer of towels (Figure 10.1). Treatment duration is usually 20–30 minutes. Electric heating pads and pads that circulate hot water are also forms of superficial heat. Infrared radiation is a seldom-utilized modality of superficial heating. It does have the advantage of being able to provide superficial heat to large surface areas, but disadvantages include skin drying and dermal photoaging.[8]

10.2.3 Deep Heat

Ultrasound (US) is the most often utilized modality for delivering deep heat. Vibrating quartz crystals from within the US applicator emit current with ultrasonic frequency. This process is a reverse piezoelectric effect. Body tissues then absorb the high-frequency acoustic energy which leads to molecular vibration with resultant conversion to thermal energy. Heat gradients are most prominent at tissue interfaces, especially between bone and soft tissue. US is administered by moving the applicator in a circular or longitudinal manner in port areas limited to 25 square cm[19] (Figure 10.2). Treatment duration ranges from 5 to 10 minutes per port. Proponents of US point to therapeutic benefits of heat as the mechanism of therapeutic effect. The advantage of US over other deep-heating modalities is the depth which heat can be delivered. Support in the literature is limited for the use of US in the case of low back pain.[27]

    In 1907, Franz Nagebehmidt demonstrated the deep-heating effects of the high-frequency current and coined the term "diathermy,"[20] which is a

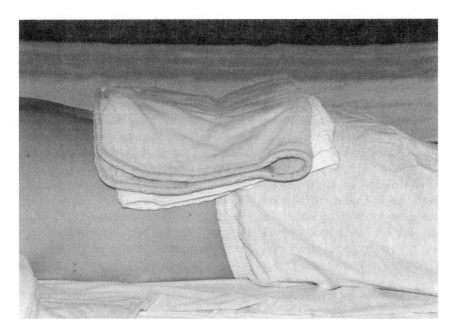

Figure 10.1 Superficial heat applied to the lumbar region with a hydrocollator pack which is indirectly placed upon the skin on a layer of towels.

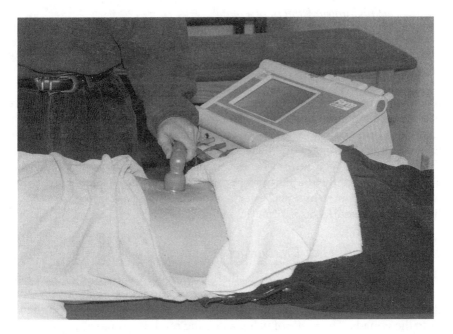

Figure 10.2 Ultrasound applied to the lumbar region.

synonym for deep heat. The first diathermy machines were both cumbersome and noisy; however, despite these drawbacks, by 1910 they were widely available as a therapeutic modality. Present day electromagnetic diathermies include shortwave diathermy (SWD) and microwave diathermy (MWD). The use of both of these modalities has essentially been eclipsed by US but for historical purposes they will be mentioned here.

In 1928, a SWD machine was developed which delivered a three-meter wave at 400 watts.[20] A lack of appropriate precautions and its overzealous use often resulted in severe burns. This lead to continuing design modifications. Even today, only the patient's perception of pain governs the dosimetry during treatment.[5] In 1954, longwave diathermy could no longer be used in treatment. The FCC currently limits the medical use of SWD to three frequencies in a range from 13.56MHz to 40.68MHz. Treatments last 20 to 30 minutes. Perspiration and metals such as jewelry can cause focal heating and burns. Pacemakers and pregnancy are both contraindications to receiving SWD.

In 1946, the extremely high frequency microwave was introduced by Frank H. Krusen and associates as a therapeutic heating modality.[16] MWD ranges in frequency from 915 MHz to 2456 MHz. Tissues with high water content absorb more energy and are selectively heated;[19] therefore, effusions and fluid-filled cavities should be avoided. Other contraindications include metal implants, pacemakers, skeletal immaturity, pregnancy, and exposure to reproductive organs.[13, 19]

10.2.4   Physiologic Effects of Heat

The direct physiological effects of heat include increases in vasodilatation and the inflammatory process as well as increases in cellular metabolic rate and collagen extensibility.[19] The therapeutic temperature range is narrow, from 40° to 45°C, with potential tissue damage occurring above 45°C. The biologic responses to heat are influenced by many factors including the source of heat, its depth and time of application, as well as the rate and area dimensions to which the heat is applied. All of these factors must be considered when selecting a therapeutic heat source. The thermal insulation quality of the subcutaneous fat limits the depth of heating by superficial thermal agents. The use of the diathermies permits the targeting of deeper structures where the direct physiological effects of heat are exerted and nerve conduction velocity is reduced resulting in analgesia.

10.2.5   General Heat Precautions

Heat should not be applied to anesthetic regions or to an obtunded patient. It should be avoided in the presence of an inadequate vascular supply or in the presence of a hemorrhagic diathesis as well as directly over a malignancy or to the gonads. The merit of using a heating modality must always be carefully considered in the context of pregnancy. Electromagnetic radiation should never be exposed to a gravid uterus. Ultrasound can exacerbate radiculopathic symptoms[11] and its application should be avoided over a laminectomy site. Excessive superficial heating can produce the epidermal reaction of skin hyperpigmentation known as erythema ab igne.

10.2.6   Historical Perspective of Therapeutic Cryotherapy

In 1850, evaporative cooling by ether was introduced by Vollemier.[20] In 1855, William Cullar produced artificial ice by passing water over nitrous ether and by 1885 artificial ice was widely available in the U.S.[12] For many years, cryotherapy has been employed in the treatment of acute soft tissue injuries. Its ready availability and ease of application are among its greatest therapeutic assets.[23]

10.3   Therapeutic Cryotherapy

Vasoconstriction is the mechanism by which cryotherapy imparts most of its therapeutic benefit. In so doing, the process of inflammation is compromised and edema is minimized which leads to the desired goal of decreased pain.[32] Cold application also reduces cellular metabolism, reduces nerve conduction velocity, decreases collagen extensibility, and decreases muscle contractibility. The result of these effects is to increase the pain threshold. Cryotherapy is usually applied for only several minutes and can take many forms such as topical ice (Figure 10.3), ice massage, commercially available cold packs, and

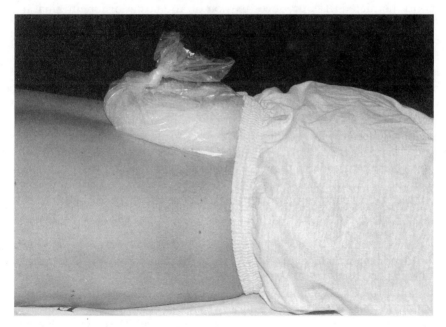

Figure 10.3   Ice pack applied to the lumbar region.

topical sprays.[19] Treatment of the paralumbar musculature, however, requires a more prolonged exposure of 20 to 30 minutes to ensure adequately deep cooling.[1] Cryotherapy is typically utilized in the acute phase of an injury but is also applied after exercise and is somewhat more effective in treating chronic conditions.[17]

10.3.1 Physiologic Effects of Cold and General Cold Precautions

Most of the undue responses to cryotherapy are related to hypersensitivity reactions including classical cold urticaria with an excessive release of histamine-like substances producing urticaria, erythema, pruritus, and in the extreme case, even anaphylaxis. Other hypersensitivity syndromes have also been described including reactions to the presence of cold hemolysins and agglutinins and reactions to the presence of cryoglobulins.[14] Such dramatic systemic complications are extremely rare in the context of localized topical application of cryotherapy.

10.4 Traction

The goal of lumbar traction is to distract the lumbar vertebra for therapeutic purposes. The theoretical effects of traction on the spine are numerous: diminishes disc protrusion, enlarges intervertebral foramen, separates intervertebral joints, stretches tight and painful joint capsules, releases entrapped synovial membranes, frees adherent nerve roots, produces central vacuum to reduce herniated disc, produces tension on the posterior longitudinal ligament which aids in reduction of disc herniation, and relaxes muscle spasm.[33] Manual traction can be applied to the lumbar spine in many positions. The recumbent, sitting, supine, prone, and standing positions are all possible. Inversion traction can also be performed but is much less specific to the lumbar region. Gravity traction utilizes a thoracic harness to suspend the patient while gravity distracts the lumbar spine. Mechanical traction can also be performed with a specifically designed traction table upon which the patient lies supine with hips and knees flexed (Figure 10.4). The upper torso is stabilized while a harness applied to the pelvis mechanically distracts the lumbar spine. The traction can be intermittent or continuous and the magnitude of force applied can be adjusted. Several prospective studies have concluded that traction is not efficacious in the treatment of lumbar spinal conditions.[6, 9]

10.5 Electrotherapy

Electrotherapy can be applied in many forms to the low back region. Transcutaneous electrical nerve stimulation (TENS), high-voltage galvanic stimulation (HVGS), interferential current stimulation (ICS), and iontophoresis are examples.

TENS is a noninvasive and relatively simple technique which has been employed in the management of chronic low back pain (Figure 10.5). The ini-

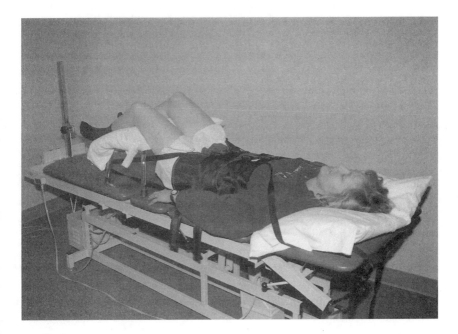

Figure 10.4 A lumbar traction table in use.

tial interest in TENS application was peaked by Wall and Sweet when they used this modality as a source of tactile stimulation to modulate pain in accord with Melzack and Wall's "Pain Gate Control Theory."[31] Kerr subsequently implicated tactile stimulation in his central inhibitory balance theory.[15] Two mechanisms have been suggested for the efficacy of TENS therapy. The first suggests that TENS inhibits pain transmission by closing a central pain gate[25] and the second implicates the release of endogenous analgesic endorphins and enkephalins.[28]

Although the mechanism of TENS action is not clearly understood, it is acknowledged that the response to treatment will vary with stimulation frequency, pulse, and intensity. The frequency of stimulation output may vary from four to eight Hz. Current intensity is initially increased to an unpleasant level and then reduced to a level of tolerance. Attempting to utilize TENS in a standardized protocol with predetermined electrode placement and frequency of stimulation is often less effective than selecting optimal parameters of stimulation individualized to the treatment session.[21]

TENS generates low-voltage stimulation which varies in frequency and the stimulation can be delivered in a pulsatile or continuous fashion. Although its definitive mechanism of action remains uncertain, some proposed theories include: the gate theory of pain, modulation of endorphins and enkephalins, and central biasing of the midbrain.[4] Opinions vary greatly regarding the efficacy of TENS therapy. Some maintain that benefit does not exceed that of placebo,[7] others believe that benefit is temporary,[24] and still

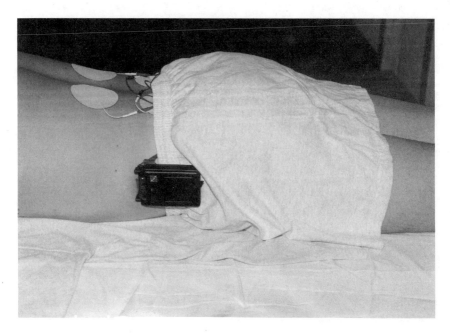

Figure 10.5   Transcutaneous electrical nerve stimulation (TENS) applied to the lumbar region.

others purport that TENS therapy is useful if used in conjunction with a multifaceted treatment program.[18] Improper electrode placement may compromise optimal response to TENS therapy.[22] The essential consideration regarding TENS therapy is that no therapeutic benefit can be expected beyond that which is derived from decreasing the pain experience.

HVGS as its name implies delivers high voltage stimulation which permits deeper tissue penetration of current and minimizes cutaneous effects. Therapeutic effects are thought to involve direct nerve fiber stimulation as well as indirectly altering blood flow and as a result edema is decreased and pain is modulated.[26]

ICS therapy delivers two medium-frequency currents that cross one another perpendicularly from two sets of electrodes which are positioned to surround the painful region in the low back (Figure 10.6). The crossing currents are set at different frequencies and it is proposed that deeper stimulation can be achieved at the point where the dissimilar currents intersect.[26] The therapeutic effects are thought to be similar to those in HVGS.

Iontophoresis is a process by which electrotherapy is utilized to direct charged particles transcutaneously (Figure 10.7). The goal is to deliver an agent, usually a corticosteroid, to the sight of inflammation in a noninvasive fashion. The fundamental question of whether or not iontophoresis can actually transport corticosteroids transcutaneously is still debated[3, 10] and

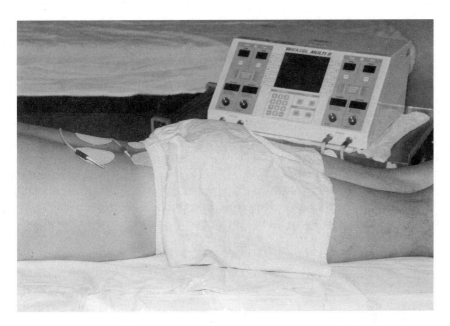

Figure 10.6   Interferential current stimulation applied to the lumbar region.

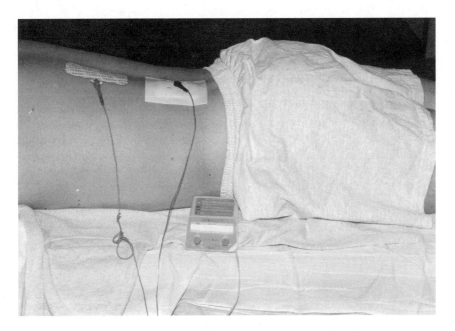

Figure 10.7   Iontophoresis applied to the lumbar region.

detractors suggest that the actual therapeutic benefit may be derived from the electrotherapy component of this modality. Most successes with iontophoresis have involved application to the limbs and there is a paucity of evidence to support the use of iontophoresis in the treatment of low back pain.

10.6 Acupuncture

The National Institute of Health published a position statement which concluded that acupuncture may be useful as an adjunct treatment or an acceptable alternative or be included in a comprehensive management program for low back pain.[30] The introduction of acupuncture into the choice of treatment modalities readily available to the American public is in its early stages. The therapeutic mechanism of action remains somewhat elusive relative to western scientific standards.

10.7 Summary

Therapeutic modalities should not be considered curative interventions. Their use, however, may facilitate a more advanced level of rehabilitation. Heating modalities, for instance, could be used on the lumbar region to increase soft tissue elasticity in order to facilitate lumbar traction. This foundation may then enable the institution of supervised rudimentary exercises that could subsequently be progressed to an active and independent exercise program. The reputation of physical agent modalities may have been tainted by practitioners who rely solely or largely on their use for the treatment of low back pain. Such treatment strategies usually lead to suboptimal outcomes. Combining physical modalities with a few specific exercises proved equally effective in treating low back pain in comparison to a progressively graded exercise program. Both approaches were superior to a self-directed walking program.[29] This suggests that physical agent modalities have a role in the treatment of LBP if they are used in the context of a multifaceted treatment program including exercise. Therapeutic modalities will likely always play a role in the treatment of low back pain. Further quality research is certainly necessary, however, to clarify this role.

All photos in Chapter 10 courtesy of Cheryl Ertelt.

10.8 References

1. Bierman, W., Friedlander, M. The penetrative effect of cold. *Arch. Phys. Ther.* 21:585, 1940.
2. Bigelow, H. R. *An International Symposium On Electrotherapeutics*, London, n.p., 1902.
3. Chantraine, A., Ludy, J. P., Berger, D. Is cortisone iontophoresis possible? *Arch. Phys. Med. Rehabil.* 67:38–40, 1986.

4. Cheng, R., Pomeranz, B. Electroacupuncture analgesic could be mediated by at least two pain relieving mechanisms: endorphin and nonendorphin systems. *Life Sci.* 25:1957–1962.
5. DeLisa, J. A. *Rehabilitation Medicine: Principals and Practice,* 2nd ed. Philadelphia: Lippincott, 1993.
6. Deyo, R. Conservative therapy for low back pain, distinguishing useful from useless therapy. *JAMA,* 250:1057–1062, 1983.
7. Deyo, R., Walsh, N., Martin, D. et al. A controlled trial of transcutaneous electrical nerve stimulation and exercise for chronic low back pain, *N. Engl. J. of Med.* 322:1627–1634, 1990.
8. Dover, J. S., Phillips, T. J., Arndt, K. A. Cutaneous effects and therapeutic uses of heat with emphasis on infrared radiation. *J. Am. Acad. Dermatol.* 20:278–286, 1989.
9. Frymoyer, J. Back pain and sciatica. *N. Engl. J. of Med.* 318:291–300, 1988.
10. Glass, J., Stephen, R., Jacobson, S. The quantity and distribution of radiolabeled dexamethasone delivered to tissue by iontophoresis, *Int. J. Dermatol.* 9:519–525, 1980.
11. Gnatz, S. M. Increased radicular pain due to therapeutic ultrasound applied to the back. *Arch. Phys. Med. Rehabil.* 70:493, 1989.
12. Henderson, A. R. John Gorrie, M.D. 1803–1855, Pioneer of air conditioning and refrigeration. *JAMA.* 185:330, 1963.
13. Jones, S. L. Electromagnetic field interference and cardiac pacemakers. *Phys. Ther.* 56:1013–1018, 1976.
14. Juhlin, L., Shelley, W. B. Role of mast cell and basophil in cold urticaria with associated systemic reactions. *JAMA.* 117:371, 1961.
15. Kerr, F. W. L. Pain: A central inhibitory balance theory. *Mayo Clin. Proc.* 50:685, 1975.
16. Krusen, F. H. Samuel Hyde Memorial Lecture: Medical Applications of Microwave Diathermy. *Proc. Roy. Soc. Med.* 43:641, August 1950.
17. Landen, B. R. Heat or cold for the relief of low back pain? *Phys. Ther.* 47:1126, 1967.
18. Langlay, G., Sheppeard, H., Johnson, M. et al. The analgesic effects of transcutaneous electrical nerve stimulation and placebo in chronic pain patients. A double-blind noncrossover comparison. *Rheumatol. Int.* 4:119–123, 1984.
19. Lehman, J. F. *Therapeutic Heat And Cold,* 4th ed. Baltimore: Williams & Wilkins, 1990.
20. Licht, S. H., Kamentz. *Therapeutic Heat And Cold,* 2nd ed. New Haven, n.p. 1965.
21. Loeser, J. D., Black, R. D., Christman, A. Relief of pain by transcutaneous stimulation. *Neurosurgery* 42:308, 1975.
22. Manheimer, J. Electrode placements for transcutaneous electrical nerve stimulation. *Phys. Ther.* 58(12):1455–1462, 1978.
23. McMaster, W. C. A literary review on ice therapy in injuries. *Am. J. Sports Med.* 3:124, 1977.
24. Melzack, R., Vetere, P., Finch, L. Transcutaneous electrical nerve stimulation for low back pain. A comparison of TENS and massage for pain and range-of-motion. *Phys. Ther.* 4:489–493, 1983.
25. Meyerson, B. A. Electrostimulation procedures: Effects, presumed rational, and possible mechanisms, in *Advances in Pain Research and Therapy, vol. 5,* Bonica, J. J., Lindbloom, U., and Iggo, A. New York: Raven Press, 495–534, 1983.

26. Reitman, C., Esses, S. Conservative options in the management of spinal disorders, part I, bed rest, mechanical, and energy-transfer therapies. 109–116, 1995.

27. Santiesteban, A. The role of physical agents in treatment of spine pain. *Clin. Orthop. Relat. Res.* 179:24–30, 1983.

28. Sjolund, B. H., Eriksonn, B. E. The influence of nalaxone on analgesia produced by peripheral conditioning stimulation. *Brain Res.* 173:295, 1979.

29. Torstensen, T. A., Ljunggren, A. E., Meen, H. D. et al. Efficacy and costs of medical exercise therapy, conventional physiotherapy, and self-exercise in patients with chronic low back pain: A pragmatic, randomized, single-blinded, controlled trial with one-year follow-up. *Spine* 23(23):2616–2624, 1998.

30. U.S. Department of Health and Human Services, NIH Consensus Statement: Acupuncture, vol. 15(5), Nov. 3–5, 1997.

31. Wall, P. D., Sweet, W. H. Temporary abolition of pain in man. *Science,* 155:108, 1967.

32. Warren, C. Use of heat and cold in treatment of common musculoskeletal disorders, in *Management of Common Musculoskeletal Disorders Physical Therapy Principals and Methods,* Kessler, R., Hertling D., eds. Philadelphia: Harper & Row, 115–127, 1983.

33. White, A. A., Panjabi, M. M. *Clinical Biomechanics of the Spine,* 2nd ed. Philadelphia: Lippincott, 432, 1990.

chapter eleven

Lumbosacral Orthotics

Agnes Soriano Wallbom, M.D.
Andrew J. Haig, M.D.

11.1   Overview

At a hotel, the housekeeping staff wear discreet black straps around their waists. An elderly man in a nursing home daily dons his white corset with metal stays, but he hasn't had back pain for years.

What place do orthoses have in the management of spinal disorders? Do they accomplish their intended purpose? Is their use justified? In the industrial world the answers to these questions are important. Discussions about orthotic management have an impact on primary, secondary, and tertiary prevention of back pain. As we will see, intelligent decisions in these areas include a number of factors.

We will begin with a basic review of the common clinical uses of orthoses. Contraindications are seldom discussed, but need to be understood. Unfortunately, there is very little clinical research on the efficacy of orthoses, so the discussion must delve into theoretical arguments. Here we will review the basic types of orthoses, biomechanical studies, and other considerations in their use. Finally, given the gaps in our knowledge about the use of orthoses, we can still make intelligent decisions, especially regarding prevention, when cost models are brought into play. One such model is presented.

11.2   Clinical Utilization

The question arises as to when lumbosacral orthoses (LSOs) are clinically indicated. There is not much in the scientific literature that documents specific clinical indications for (LSO) duration of use or indications for cessation of use.[1] LSOs are part of a therapeutic armamentarium[2, 3] the goal of which is to

0-8493-0089-4/00/$0.00+$.50
© 2000 by CRC Press LLC

decrease pain, increase functional capacity, decrease disability, and prevent future back injury. They are prescribed in a variety of conditions including internal disc derangements, herniated nucleus pulposus, vertebral body fracture, spondylolysis with instability and listhesis, spinal stenosis, and postoperative use after decompressive surgery.[4] However, the efficacy of an LSO remains unproven for the majority of lumbar spine conditions.

An LSO may be used for spinal segmental instability.[5–10] One example would be to prescribe an LSO for patients with a spondylolisthesis complaining of back pain with movement. The goal is to decrease the movement and, therefore, pain. Because of this, most clinicians would recommend a rigid orthosis to minimize movement. The length of use will depend upon when the patient becomes asymptomatic and/or when the spine is deemed stable. The orthosis can also be used as a preoperative trial to determine whether a patient's symptoms are improved with immobilization prior to fixation surgery. The major drawback to using a rigid orthosis is the discomfort to the patient because of the rigidity. The patient may feel that donning the orthosis is cumbersome. Once on, the orthosis can alter the patient's body perception as the orthosis adds an additional layer. This produces bulk and retains heat. In addition, varying positions and movements of the patient may diminish its intended effect of stabilization.

An orthosis may be prescribed for temporary use. An abdominal sling or soft neoprene lumbosacral corset is sometimes prescribed for short duration for symptomatic treatment resulting from the altered biomechanics of an obese individual who is becoming more active after a sedentary lifestyle. In addition, patients with a mild scoliosis may wear an orthosis for symptomatic relief if it can increase function such as sitting tolerance.

11.3   Contraindications

Most clinicians will agree that the use of an LSO for extended periods of time is not appropriate. One argument for this is the expectation that the wearer will become both physically and psychologically dependent upon the orthosis. Although there are studies stating that the use of an orthosis does not produce muscle atrophy and deconditioning,[11–13] many clinicians adhere to the idea that prolonged use weakens the back and abdominal muscles. Psychological dependence may be interpreted by the patient as validation of a disability. Clinicians need to be aware of this in selectively prescribing orthotic management. This must be seen as a treatment for a specific condition or must not make a patient more disabled than their baseline presentation. It is insufficient to prescribe a nonrigid orthosis in the presence of significant instability. It is important to appropriately match the underlying anatomical structure and biomechanics with the type of external support.

Safety concerns regarding the use of an LSO are important. Orthoses are relatively contraindicated in persons who work around machinery. Lumbar belts with loose straps, for example, may cause injury. Likewise, if someone requires much flexibility in their duties, it might be unsafe to prescribe a rigid immobilizing orthosis. To do so may lead to an increased risk of falling while performing one's regular job duties. In a hot work environment, the heat retaining property of a rigid plastic orthosis, for example, may make a patient more noncompliant. If the patient remains compliant, he may become more prone to dehydration as heat retention leads to more sweating. Orthoses should be avoided in patients with uncontrolled hypertension, aortic aneurysm, or other disorders adversely affected by increased intra-abdominal pressure. Finally, it is inappropriate to prescribe an orthosis for someone who clearly states they would be unable or unwilling to comply with the prescription.

11.4 Actions of Lumbosacral Orthoses

11.4.1 Rigidity

Lumbosacral orthoses are based on varying degrees of rigidity or flexibility, postural control, and load relieving effect. The rigidity of an orthosis is based on the three-point pressure principle. There are two counterforces applied at superior and inferior aspects of an orthosis with an oppositely directed third force in the middle on the opposite side. If the third force is anterior, the orthosis promotes flexion such as with the Raney jacket. If posterior, the orthosis promotes extension as with Dr. Jewett's design (Figure 11.1). Superior support is located inferior to the xiphoid process and the scapulae. Inferior support is located superior to the pelvis and proximal to the greater trochanters at the level of the midsacrum.

11.4.2 Immobilization

Immobilization consists of two types: segmental or gross. Segmental immobilization is the elimination of motion of a particular motion segment and is accomplished by a rigid orthosis or internal or external fixation. These are used in the management of fractures, fracture dislocations, spondylitis, and degenerative or postoperative instability. Gross restriction is the decrease in range of motion in one or more of the three planes to allow the patient to function in a pain-free range.

In a study by Norton and Brown which used Kirschner wires to measure motion, orthoses provided little intersegmental spinal immobilization.[14] The immobilization of intersegmental motion as measured by radiographs varies significantly dependent on the type of orthosis. One radiographic study showed that the TLSO had no stabilizing effect on sagittal intervertebral translation.[15] The TLSO with hip and thigh extensions showed a small decrease in sagittal mobility.[16] A corset-type orthosis decreased intersegmental motion by 30% at all levels. A Raney jacket and a similar cast decreased motion by 66% in the midlumbar region. A cast decreased motion by 92% at L4–5 and at L5–S1.[17]

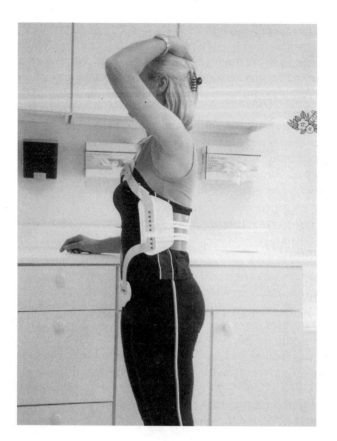

Figure 11.1   Jewett hyperextension orthosis. Photo courtesy of Toenges Orthotics and Prosthetics.

The effect of immobilization of gross motion also varies with the types of orthosis. The TLSO, LSO with anterior-posterior control, and corset-type LSO decreased motion up to 20% in flexion and 45% in extension. Limitation of lateral bending may be accomplished by adding lateral longitudinal bars. The effectiveness of these bars is a function of their rigidity and the quality of the interface at the thorax and pelvis. This may be effective but poorly tolerated by the patient.[14] Using plastic foam interface materials may create a more tolerable TLSO. The lumbosacral corset restricted lateral bending by 29%, LSO, anterior-posterior control, 45%; and TLSO, body jacket type, 49%.[18] A recent study by Tuong demonstrated that an LSO decreases vertebral mobility and discal deformations mainly at L1–3 but increases it at inferior levels.[19]

Axial rotation of the lumbosacral spine averaged 6 degrees during standing and 1 to 5 degrees during walking. In Lumsden's study lumbosacral orthoses actually increased axial rotation in some subjects.[20] The trunk and pelvis are similar to an oval cylinder with the spine lending support. Fixation depends on the fit between the orthosis and bony prominences. However, skin and soft tissue—the loose layers between the skeleton and orthosis— make fixation by the orthosis difficult. Superiorly, the thorax provides a large bony surface area. Inferiorly, the pelvis has a much smaller surface area. Therefore, incorporating a hip joint and thigh cuff for fixation may be more mechanically efficient but cause the patient to be more uncomfortable.

11.4.3   Load-Relieving Effects

Normally, the anterior abdominal muscles (transverse and oblique) increase intra-abdominal pressure. The literature varies concerning whether corsets increase intra-abdominal pressure and whether increased intra-abdominal pressure has a load-relieving effect on the spine.[21, 22, 27] Some authors have reported that during forward bending, there is a reduction in intradiscal pressure while wearing an orthosis.[23–25]

11.4.4   Other Effects

Orthoses may increase warmth to the trunk muscles thereby leading to more relaxation. There is a reported placebo effect and skin warming.[26] Skin temperature does not increase significantly, though, unless the orthosis is thick and padded.[27]

11.5   Types of Lumbosacral Orthoses

11.5.1   Lumbosacral Orthosis, Corset-Type

A commonly prescribed spinal orthosis is a lumbosacral corset made of a dacron/cotton material (Figure 11.2). It is washable and closes with a snap or zipper front and buckle or Velcro sides. The typical corset has four to six inches of adjustment in the side panels. The orthosis comes with removable stays for use in pockets along the length of the paraspinal muscles. These stays may or may not be used. If used, it is imperative that they be shaped properly to accommodate the patient's anatomy and function. The patient is instructed to close the orthosis from inferior to superior with the most inferior strap between the iliac crest and the trochanter. The orthosis should not migrate when the patient sits.

11.5.2   Semirigid Orthoses

There are two types of semirigid lumbosacral orthoses consisting of metal with a leather or vinyl cover and/or thermoplastic (Figure 11.3). The LSO, anterior-posterior control, consists of two paraspinal bars connected to pelvic and thoracic bands posteriorly and a "pie pan" abdominal support anteriorly. The LSO with anterior-posterior-lateral control is similar but has lateral bars and normally a full-corset front. The LSO with anterior-posterior-lateral

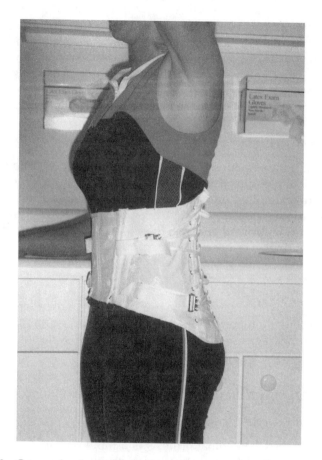

Figure 11.2 Canvas lumbosacral corset with stays. Photo courtesy of Toenges Orthotics and Prosthetics.

control tends to restrict the thoraco-lumbar spine but increases lumbosacral movement with moderate to vigorous activity.[14] The disadvantages of semi-rigid orthoses are that they are less comfortable than the corset type and are more expensive. Their advantage is that they may be slightly cooler than the corset. They are fitted according to hip size and the length from the sacrococcygeal junction to the inferior angle of the inferior scapular border.

11.5.3 Industrial Lumbar Support

The traditional belt used in the work force to prevent injuries is usually made of fabric and elastic with Velcro/buckle closures (Figure 11.4). Sometimes there are flexible metal or plastic stays or a plastic back panel for additional stabilization. Additional features may include adjustable side pull straps and/or an air bladder. This is fitted to an individual's waist size. The disadvantage of this support is that it is difficult to stabilize over the iliac crests.

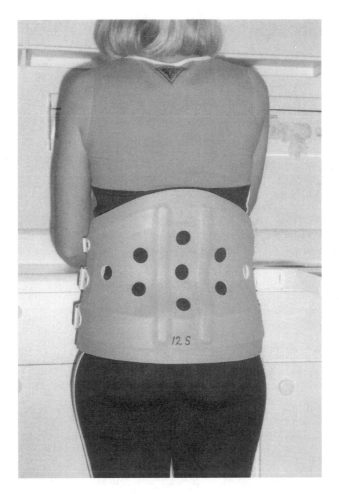

Figure 11.3 Semirigid lumbosacral orthosis. Photo courtesy of Toenges Orthotics and Prosthetics.

Currently, studies of lumbosacral supports have been done with a wider front panel.[25]

In order to maintain placement of an LSO the orthosis may be fitted with peroneal straps or with elastic athletic shorts. This is a solution to keep the orthosis in place which may aid in stabilizing the hips and pelvis as well. These components must be custom-fitted.

11.6   Industrial Economic Factors

Decisions regarding the use of spinal orthoses in industrial settings require analyses which go beyond discussions of effectiveness. In the industrial setting, a number of practical, political, psychosocial, and economic factors come into play. Primary prevention is an example.

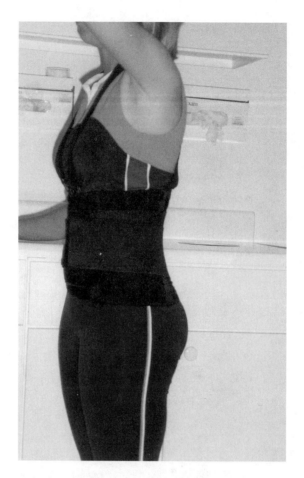

Figure 11.4   Industrial lumbosacral corset. Photo courtesy of Toenges Orthotics and Prosthetics.

Acknowledging that there is not enough factual information to confidently predict any preventive effect of orthotic management, the occupational health physician can still make some decisions regarding their use, based on modeling of costs and intelligent guessing. We will calculate the effect based on realistic but fabricated data.

Table 11.1 provides information on a hypothetical "XYZ Corp." In this situation, if we assume that corsets prevent 100% of back claims, at the most they would provide a 47% savings. Given that the vast majority of back complaints are not related to a specific lifting event, and that corsets cannot be expected to prevent slips, trips, falls, pain from outside of work, psychogenic pain disorders, and secondary gain issues, it would be very impressive if corsets prevented even 20% of complaints. Even here, the numbers suggest that this company would lose a significant amount of money. While the numbers may be quite different with different industries, different worker com-

Table 11.1 Theoretical economic considerations.

	XYZ Corporation
Number of employees	1,000
Back injury incidence/year	5%
Number of injuries/year	50
Average cost per injury	<u>$10,000</u>
Total cost for back pain/year	$500,000
Corsets per employee/year	2
Employee turnover	10%
Number of corsets needed	2,200
Cost of one corset	<u>$100</u>
Total material costs:	$220,000
Orientation and implementation[a]	$44,000
Employee health/upper management time	$?
Union/management issues	$?
Increase in awareness of pain[b]	<u>$?</u>
Total cost for corsets	$264,000
Cases prevented	Savings (cost)
100%	$236,000
80%	$136,000
50%	[−$14,000]
20%	[−$164,000]

(a) 1 hour per employee orientation + 1 hour per employee implementation, enforcement of rules, etc. × $20.00/hour.

(b) Surveys show that most persons have a backache in any given week, but most do not report it or seek care. Employees who are made to pay attention to the medical issues regarding their back on a daily basis may experience more concerns and increase health care utilization.

pensation statutes, and other variations in cost and savings, the illustration points out that economic incentives to use corsets in prevention may be surprisingly few.

The "soft" concerns are equally important. It is likely that an employer's requirement that corsets be worn will not be taken lightly by employees or by their union representatives. Enforcement of compliance with rules regarding corsets involves the same energy and expense as enforcement of ear protection and eye protection rules. It costs money to monitor employees, to send them back to put on their corsets, and to discipline them when they do not comply. Some employees (for example, pregnant women) should not be wearing certain corsets.

11.7 Summary

While many physicians commonly prescribe lumbosacral orthoses for chronic lower back pain,[28] future studies are needed to address the efficacy of corsets in specific clinical settings. One hypothesis could be: Does a lumbosacral corset decrease pain and improve function in those with chronic lower back pain secondary to degenerative disc disease? The challenges of prospective clinical research studies would include defining inclusion and exclusion criteria (diagnoses, similar signs and symptoms, "red flags"), outcome measurements (function, pain), and intervention (LSO type, frequency and duration of use). However, at this time there is limited data to support the use of lumbosacral corsets for the majority of low back disorders in the occupational setting.

11.8   References

1. Pope, M. H., Fryomoyer, J. W., and Andersson, G. *Occupational Low Back Pain,* New York: Praeger, 191, 1984.
2. Coxhead, C. E., Mead, T. W., Inskip, H., North, W. R. S., and Troup, J. D. G. Multicentre trial of physiotherapy in the management of sciatic symptoms, *Lancet,* 1, 1065, 1981.
3. Pope, M. H., Phillips, R. B., Haugh, L. D., Hsieh, C. J., MacDonald, L., and Haldeman, S. A prospective randomized three-week trial of spinal manipulation, transcutaneous muscle stimulation, massage, and corset in the treatment of subacute low back pain, *Spine,* 19, 2571, 1994.
4. Nachemson, A. Orthotic treatment for injuries and diseases of the spinal column, *Arch. Phys. Med. Rehabil.,* 1, 11, 1987.
5. Ahlgren, A. The use of lumbosacral corsets prescribed for low back pain, *Prosthet. Orthot. Int.,* 6, 79, 1982.
6. Million, R., Nilsen, H., Jayson, M. I. V., and Baker, R. D. Evaluation of low back pain and assessment of lumbar corsets with and without back supports, *Ann. Rheum. Dis.,* 40, 449, 1981.
7. Million, R., Hall, W., Nilsen, K., Baker, R. D., and Jayson, M. I. V. Assessment of the progress of the back-pain patients, *Spine,* 7, 204, 1982.
8. Larsson, U., Cholers, U., Lindstrom, A., Lind, G., Nachemson, A., Nilsson, B., and Roslund, J. Autotraction for treatment of lumbago scientica. A multicentre controlled investigation, *Acta. Orthop. Scand.,* 51, 791, 1980.
9. Micheli, L. J., Hall, J. E., and Miller, M. E. Use of the modified Boston brace for back injuries in athletes, *Am. J. Sports Med.,* 8, 351, 1980.
10. Willner, F. Effect of a rigid brace on back pain, *Acta. Orthop. Scand.,* 56, 40, 1985.
11. Walsh, N. E. and Schwartz, R. K. The influence of prophylactic orthoses on abdominal strength and low back injury in the workplace, *Am. J. Phys. Med. Rehabil.,* 69, 245, 1990.
12. Nachemson, A. and Lindh, M. Measurement of abdominal and back muscle strength with and without low back pain, *Scand. J. Rehab. Med.,* 1, 60, 1969.
13. Holstrom, E. and Moritz, U. Effects of lumbar belts on trunk muscle strength and endurance: a follow-up of construction workers, *J. Spinal Disord.,* 5, 260, 1992.
14. Norton, P. L. and Brown, T. The immobilizing efficiency of back braces: their effect on posture in motion of the lumbosacral spine, *JBJS,* 39(A), 111, 1957.
15. Axelsson, P., Johnsson, R., and Stromqvist, B. Effect of lumbar orthosis on intervertebral mobility. A roentgen stereophotogrammetric analysis, *Spine,* 17, 678, 1992.

16. Axelsson, P., Johnsson, R., and Stromqvist, B. Lumbar orthosis with unilateral hip immobilization: effect on intervertebral mobility determined by roentgen stereophotogrammetric analysis, *Spine*, 18, 876, 1993.

17. Fidler, M. W. and Plasmans, C. M. T. The effect of four types of support on the segmental mobility of the lumbosacral spine, *JBJS*, 65(A), 943, 1983.

18. Lantz, S. A. and Schultz, A. B. Lumbar spine orthosis wearing. I. Restriction of gross body motions, *Spine*, 11, 834, 1986.

19. Tuong, N. H., Dansereau, J., Maurais, G., and Herrera, R. Three-dimensional evaluation of lumbar orthosis effects on spinal behavior, *J. Rehabil. Res. Dev.*, 35, 34, 1998.

20. Lumsden, R. M. and Morris, J. M. An in vivo study of axial rotation and immobilization at the lumbosacral joint, *JBJS*, 50A, 1591, 1968.

21. Morris, J. M., Lucas, D. B. and Bresler, B. Role of the trunk in stability of the spine, *JBJS*, 43A, 327, 1961.

22. Garg, A. Manual material handling: The science, in *Musculoskeletal Disorders in the Workplace Principles and Practice*, Nordin, M., Andersson, G., Pope, M., eds., Chicago: Mosby, 1997.

23. Nachemson, A., Schultz, A., and Andersson, G. Mechanical effectiveness studies of lumbar spine orthoses, *Scand. J. Rehabil. Med.*, 9(S), 139, 1983.

24. Nachemson, A. Advances in low back pain, *Clin. Orthop. Res.*, 200, 266, 1985.

25. Nachemson, A. and Morris, J. M. In vivo measurements of intradiscal pressure, *JBJS*, 46A, 1077, 1964.

26. Dixon, A. S., Owen-Smith, B. D., and Harrison, R. A. Cold-sensitive, nonspecific, low back pain (a comparative trial of treatment), *Clin. Trials J.*, 9, 16, 1972.

27. Grew, N. D. and Deane, G. The physical effect of lumbar spine supports, *Pros. Orth. Int.*, 6, 79, 1982.

28. Perry, J. The use of external support in the treatment of low back pain, *JBJS*, 52A, 1440, 1970.

chapter twelve

Operative Intervention for Lumbar Spine Disorders

John I. Williams, M.D.
Thomas S. Whitecloud, M.D.

12.1   Overview

The role of the spinal surgeon in the management of lumbar spinal problems has changed dramatically over the past three decades. Our understanding of lumbar spine pathology has improved, as has our ability to manage these problems both nonoperatively and operatively. The complexity of lumbar spine problems, as well as its prevalence and impact on our society, has spawned new areas of subspecialization for the care of musculoskeletal pathology.

12.2   Multidisciplinary Management of Low Back Pain

Most acute low back pain is seen first by primary care physicians, but historically the orthopaedic surgeon was responsible for managing chronic back pain. The medical and socioeconomic impact of low back problems on our society has lead to the evolution and growth of this segment of the health care arena. Due to its complexity, it has become apparent that a multidisciplinary approach is needed for the care of chronic low back pain, involving family practitioners, physiatrists, physical therapists, psychiatrists, and psychologists specializing in pain management, pain-fellowship-trained anesthesiologists, neuroradiologists, vocational rehabilitation personnel, and spinal surgeons. All bring unique talents to assist in the management of spinal problems.

Obviously, a team leader is needed to direct and coordinate the low back pain patient's care. An effective leader is one who can guide a patient through the myriad of health care personnel involved in treating spinal problems. Proper direction through this maze is the best way of obtaining the patient's short- and long-term goals in the most efficient and cost-effective manner. This task is one best performed by a physician who practices nonoperative spine care. For this reason, a physiatrist or other specialist with a strong background in musculoskeletal training is in the most effective position to direct the patient's evaluation and management within the spinal care team. A surgeon with a subspecialization in spine surgery and a commitment to nonoperative management needs to work closely with rehabilitative specialists with a comprehensive understanding of nonoperative spine management.

12.3   Surgical Evaluation

An important element is the point at which primary care of a patient is transferred from the nonoperative specialist to the surgeon. While a team approach to the management of spinal problems is critical, the spinal surgeon maintains the primary role in preoperative and intraoperative decision making. In the past, a surgical consultation was obtained when a spinal problem was not responding to the management of the primary care physician. The surgeon would then make the decision whether or not to operate. If the decision was made to operate and the patient achieved a poor result, the decision making process was restarted and the patient was either a candidate for an additional surgery or was referred to a nonsurgical specialist or primary care physician. The past several decades have proven that the pre- and postoperative rehabilitative management of patients with spinal problems is every bit as important as the surgery. For this reason, when a patient with a spinal problem has failed a course of nonoperative management and the primary decision making in the patient's care is passed from the physiatrist to the surgeon, both physicians should remain involved in the patient's management. The postoperative rehabilitative expertise that a physiatrist brings to a spinal care management team is valuable. Further benefit of a team approach to spinal problems is the shared decision making as to which patients are candidates for surgical intervention.

The final decision to operate remains the responsibility of the surgeon. Spinal problems requiring operative intervention can be broken down into two broad categories involving urgent and nonurgent problems. Urgent problems make up a small subset of the total population of people with problems. Pathology which requires urgent surgical intervention involves patients with: 1) progressive neurological deficits; 2) cauda equina syndrome; 3) lumbar trauma with instability and/or neurological deficits; 4) tumor; and 5) infection. A stable neurological deficit due to a radiculopathy is not an absolute surgical indication. For example, a foot drop from a lumbar radiculopathy may be a neurapraxic lesion which is potentially reversible and hence may respond well to nonsurgical care.

The nonurgent indication for surgery is pain. Surgical intervention for acute radicular pain is considered 6 to 8 weeks after the onset of symptoms in patients who have failed to improve with nonoperative care. A nonoperative course of management may include rest, activity modification, patient education, physical therapy, oral medications, and the use of epidural steroid injections. Patients with persistent mechanical back pain and instability may be considered for a lumbar stabilizing procedure after failing six to 12 months of aggressive nonoperative treatment.

When providing acute nonoperative care, a specific diagnosis is difficult to achieve. Low back pain is a syndrome, not a diagnosis. However, when an accurate diagnosis is obtained, the physician can provide a focused treatment plan. This plan is continually reassessed as patient management continues. This treatment plan should be reviewed with the patient so that there is a clear understanding of the natural history and prognosis of his problem. He must have realistic expectations of the long-term outlook for his condition. There must be a clear understanding of the potential benefits and risks of treatment, whether that treatment be operative or nonoperative. An informed patient involved in appropriate decision making is essential and will maximize the likelihood of success with nonsurgical and surgical treatment programs.

12.4   Surgical Intervention

When the decision is made that surgical intervention is in the patient's best interest, a precise diagnosis is required. The same two components of treatment remain critical to a positive surgical outcome. First, an unequivocal diagnosis of the patient's problem must be made, and second, patient education is required to ensure that they understand the gravity and implication of this diagnosis and that their expectations of the outcomes of surgical treatment are realistic. When a patient understands that he or she may not get back to a preinjury activity level, even if their problem is treated with an operation, they will not have unrealistic expectations. The type of operation performed should be tailored to the patient's specific diagnosis, as well as to allow the patient to realize their short- and long-term goals. Preoperative planning involves finding the safest procedure that will allow the patient to realistically achieve their goals. Larger and more extensive procedures resulting in both increased risks and recovery time, however, may be necessary in light of a patient's short- and long-term objectives.

Preoperatively, the nonoperative members of the spine team know the patient better than the surgeon. They understand the patient's character and also have a better feel for the patient's psychosocial reserves, both of which will influence the patient's postoperative rehabilitation. The patient's postoperative rehabilitation is not a passive component of his overall treatment. He requires continued intervention from both the surgeon and the physiatrist for best long-term results.

Choosing the proper surgical intervention requires a focused diagnosis. Pinpointing the origin of the patient's most significant problem, or the patient's most acute "pain generator," is the challenge before the surgeon. Multiple diagnostic tools are available to the surgeon attempting to pinpoint the origin of the patient's problem. Plain radiographs, particularly lateral flexion/extension films, will demonstrate translational pathology in the sagittal plane of the spine. An MRI will not only delineate encroachment upon the neural elements of the spine, but is also a sensitive test to identify the presence of degenerative changes within the intervertebral discs. A myelogram/CT scan remains an excellent tool in evaluating hypertrophic degenerative disease in the geriatric population or in evaluating the multi-operated spine, particularly when scoliosis is present. A bone scan may be helpful in identifying inflammation due to specific facet arthropathy. Discography remains our only test capable of identifying symptomatic degenerative intervertebral discs. Discography is considered if a patient has failed conservative treatment and is being considered for a spinal fusion. The decision to consider a fusion should be made only after all modalities of nonoperative treatment are exhausted. A discogram should be performed by an unbiased, and therefore objective, diagnostician.

The objective of spinal arthrodesis for low back pain is to decrease motion at the level of a painful motion segment. The clearest indication for spinal fusion is spinal instability as documented on the preoperative plain films. This is motion detected in the sagittal plane of the spine. Lateral flexion/extension radiographs should document greater than 3 mm of translation. Other indications for arthrodesis are: 1) iatrogenic spinal instability, an instability that occurs due to an extensive spinal decompression in which enough of the posterior elements are removed that the spine is left unstable; 2) failed back syndrome, a persistent pain and appropriate degenerative findings on imaging studies following previous surgery for either disc herniations or stenosis; 3) multiple recurrent disc herniations at the same level, which has a current recommendation that if surgery is required for a third disc herniation at the same level, then an arthrodesis should be performed; and 4) spinal arthrodesis, which may be indicated for discogenic pain documented by positive discography.[11]

The role of spinal instrumentation to facilitate arthrodesis continues to change. Zdeblick and others have shown spinal instrumentation acts to decrease the time required to achieve solid arthrodesis, as well as decrease the rate of pseudoarthrosis.[1, 8, 14] However, Turner reported no improvement in outcomes with instrumentation, and had increased risk of complications, including 8% reoperation for removal of hardware.[13] The role of anterior spinal fusion with or without posterior spinal fusion is currently under debate. There is an increased tendency to use interbody arthrodesis techniques, along with posterior instrumentation and fusion, in 1) patients who are smokers; 2) situations where there is a desire for a rapid fusion; 3) situations where there is a failure of previous posterolateral fusion; and 4) the treatment of discogenic pain as confirmed by discography.[10]

12.5   Surgical Outcomes

Reported surgical outcomes in the literature vary and are dependent on multiple factors (Figure 1). Good to excellent results have been reported following laminectomy and disc excision for routine lumbar disc herniations in 70% to 90% of patients.[3, 4, 9] These outcomes appear to be affected by the patients' workers' compensation status. Klecamp reported that lumbar discectomy patients without compensation or litigation issues had good outcomes in 81% of participants.[6] The success of lumbar surgery dropped to 50% good results in workers' compensation population, and to 23% success rate in those involved in both compensation and litigation.[7] These outcomes have been challenged by Mayer who has reported 85% return-to-work following lumbar surgery and comprehensive post-op rehabilitation.[7]

With spinal stenosis, patients with primarily leg pain can obtain excellent relief of symptoms with a decompression without fusion.[2] Reported outcomes have been as high as 92% improvement in patients with leg pain as their main complaint.[14] Tuite reported only 66% good to excellent outcome in 119 patients who underwent decompressive laminectomies without fusion for spinal stenosis.[12] Turner has reported there is no evidence to indicate that fusion improves laminectomy outcomes for uncomplicated spinal stenosis.[13]

Patients undergoing a spinal fusion for the treatment of back pain manifest variable results.[1, 8, 10, 11, 13] Outcomes were not statistically different regardless of the type of fusion procedure chosen.[10] Some authors report that instrumentation did not affect outcomes, although previously operated patients had a poorer prognosis for improvement if instrumentation was not used.[1, 14] The most common complications reported are pseudoarthrosis and chronic pain at the donor site.[13] Outcomes for lumbar fusion in the workers' compensation population are variable but generally more poor.[5, 7] Reduced outcomes were predicted by older age at the time of injury, greater percent of time on disability, longer time from injury to surgery, increased number of prior lumbar surgeries and greater number of fusion levels.[10, 11, 14]

Poor outcomes following spinal surgery can be attributed to: 1) incorrect initial diagnosis; 2) poor patient selection; 3) surgery which is not directed at the patient's most significant complaint; 4) improperly directed rehabilitation; 5) poor patient education; 6) incomplete understanding of the importance of postoperative rehabilitation; and 7) secondary gain issues with respect to workers' compensation injuries.

12.6   Summary

A team approach is critical in order to maintain a high standard of healthcare directed at spinal problems. Effective treatment—whether nonoperative or operative treatment is administered—requires an accurate diagnosis, thorough patient education to ensure realistic expectations, and a competent team of health care professionals. If surgical intervention is to be successful, a healthy interaction must continue between the patient's primary care physician, a physical medicine and rehabilitation specialist, one or more diagnosticians, and the spinal surgeon.

12.7 References

1. Buttermann, G., Garvey, T., Hunt, A. et al. Lumbar fusion results related to diagnosis, *Spine* 23, no. (1)116–127, 1998.
2. Dawson, E. and Bernbeck, J. The surgical treatment of low back pain, *Phys. Med. Rehabil. Clin. N. Am.*, 9(2), 1998.
3. Errico, T. J. Open discectomy as treatment for herniated nucleus pulposus of the lumbar spine, *Contemporary Concepts in Spine Care, N. Am. Spine Soc.*, Feb 1994:2.
4. Finneson, B. E. A lumbar disc surgery predictive scoreboard, *Spine* 3:186–187, 1978.
5. Fischgrund, J. and Montgomery, D. Diagnosis and treatment of discogenic low back pain, *Orthopaed. Rev.*, 311–318, March 1993.
6. Klecamp, J. et al. *Results of Elective Lumbar Discectomy for Workers' Compensation Patients.* San Francisco: American Academy of Orthopaedic Surgeons, 1997.
7. Mayer, T. et al. Socioeconomic outcomes of combined spine surgery and functional restoration in Worker's Compensation spinal disorders with matched controls, *Spine* 23 (5):598–606, 1998.
8. Lorenz, M. et al. A comparison of single-level fusions with and without instrumentation, *Spine* 455, 1991.
9. Spangler, D. M. Lumbar discectomy, results of a limited disc excision and selective foraminotomy, *Spine* 7:604–7, 1982.
10. Stauffer, R. K., Coventry, M. Anterior interbody lumbar spine fusion, *J. Bone Surg.* 1972; 54a:756–768.
11. Stauffer, R., Coventry, M. Posterolateral lumbar spine fusion-analysis of Mayo Clinic series, *J. Bone Joint Surg.* 172, 54a, 1195–1204.
12. Tuite, G., Stern, J., Doran, S. et al. Outcome after laminectomy for lumbar spine stenosis, *J. Neurosurg.* 81:699–706, 1994.
13. Turner, J. A., Ersek, M., Herron, L. et al. Patient outcomes after lumbar spinal fusions: A comprehensive literature synthesis, *JAMA* 268:907–911 1992.
14. Zdeblick, T. The treatment of degenerative lumbar disorders: A critical review of the literature, *Spine* 20(24s):126s–137s, 1995.

part three

Prevention

chapter thirteen

Prevention of Occupational Low Back Pain

Bryan D. Kaplansky, M.D.
Frank Y. Wei, M.D.
Mark V. Reecer, M.D.

13.1   Overview

The enormous socioeconomic impact of occupational low back pain and disability has led health care providers and industry to take a closer look at low back pain prevention. The focus on prevention strategies in the workplace by the health care industry, governmental regulatory agencies, and employers has led to a growth in the field of ergonomics. In addition to ergonomics, several other prevention strategies continue to be studied and implemented including worker selection methods, education and training techniques, exercise, risk factor modification, and orthotics. The efficacy of these prevention techniques is varied and controversial[44, 47, 65, 75] and will be reviewed in this chapter.

13.2   Prevention Principles

Prevention can take place at the primary, secondary, and tertiary levels. *Primary prevention* involves measures to prevent the occurrence of low back pain. *Secondary prevention* involves measures that attempt to reduce the prevalence of low back pain through early detection and treatment. *Tertiary prevention* involves strategies that minimize the consequences of low back pain by reducing chronic impairment and disability.

Primary prevention of low back pain in the workplace is usually the most common strategy utilized by employers. However, there is considerable overlap among the primary, secondary and tertiary prevention strategies for occupational low back pain. For example, education and training, exercise programs, risk factor modification, and ergonomic interventions can be used at the primary, secondary, and tertiary levels of prevention.

13.3   Prevention Strategies

13.3.1   Ergonomics

Ergonomics, or "human factor engineering," involves the study of the interaction between the worker and his or her environment. Ergonomists try to identify and then reduce stress factors which increase the worker's risk for injury. The goal of job design then is to match the workplace with the worker. Since "overexertion" while maneuvering objects is the most common event leading to injury in the work place,[135] job design theoretically should benefit both the employee and employer by:

1. Increasing worker safety by decreasing the risk of injury.
2. Diminishing the risk for chronic symptoms/disability for workers.
3. Keeping the worker working/matching the work tasks to the worker's capabilities.
4. Improving productivity.
5. Reducing corporate medical/disability costs.

Risk factor assessment for occupational low back pain is the first step in an ergonomic evaluation. The literature has identified several risk factors for low back pain including heavy physical work demands, frequent bending and stooping, repetitive work, static postures, sudden or unexpected movements, vibration, and job tasks that involve frequent lifting, pulling, or pushing.[4, 91] Additionally, there are psychological and social risk factors which have been linked to back pain.[15, 18, 49, 62, 109, 133] Once the risk factors for occupational low back pain are identified, the next step in an ergonomics evaluation involves job analysis.

A job analysis is a process that combines *biomechanical, physical,* and *physiologic* criteria to determine reasonable loads for workers. In addition to analyzing worker and task characteristics, the equipment, materials, work station, and environment also are assessed. *Biomechanical* analysis of a task involves: 1) the description of the action of effort (i.e., push/pull/lift); 2) determination of body posture; 3) measurement of forces applied by the worker; 4) monitoring the vertical distance between the hands and feet; 5) measurement of the frequency of an action; and 6) evaluation of the work station and environment. *Physical* analysis entails determining the amount and direction of forces applied to and by the worker during the task. *Physiologic* analysis is the assessment of the metabolic or aerobic demands of a task.

Several psychophysical and biomechanical models have been developed to facilitate the process of job analysis and job design. Psychophysical models incorporate the concept of Maximal Acceptable Weight (MAW). This value is determined by the worker's perceived exertion for various material handling tasks. Simple two-dimensional static strength and more complex three-dimensional biomechanical models are available to help determine compressive and sheer forces on the lumbar spine. Other ergonomic tools include energy expenditure and perceived stress models and The National Institute for Occupational Safety and Health Guidelines (NIOSH). Specific ergonomic design criteria describing acceptable limits for compressive force, strength, energy expenditure, heart rate, postural stress, and perceived stress have been reported based on the available models (Table 13.1).

The National Institute of Occupational Safety and Health revised the 1981[106] lifting equation in 1991[139] in an attempt to determine recommended weight limits for workers (Table 13.2). The revised lifting equation reflects a greater variety of lifting tasks. Using the NIOSH equation, a recommended weight limit is computed by determining the horizontal and vertical location of the load, the vertical travel distance of the load, the frequency and duration of the task, the angular displacement of the load, and the coupling of the load. Theoretically then, the risk of injury increases using the NIOSH equation when the horizontal distance of the hands from the body increases, the hands are close to the floor when initiating lifting, the vertical travel distance of the load to be lifted increases, the load is lifted frequently and for long periods of time, the angular displacement of the load increases and the grip is poor (Table 13.3). The ideal lifting situation based on the NIOSH equation is defined as lifting with the hands close to the body (up to 10 inches from the vertical line drawn from the ankles), lifting at a 30-inch height to a distance of up to 10 inches vertically, with a lifting frequency of once every 5 minutes or less and with the lifting duration not to exceed one hour, with no twisting, and a good grasp of the load.[44] A lifting index or an "index of relative physical stress" was also described to protect workers from hazardous loads.[139]

Table 13.1 Recommended Ergonomic Design Criteria

Criteria	Acceptable Limit
Compressive force	≤770 lb.
Strength	≥75% capable
Energy expenditure	3.1 kcal/min (whole body)
	2.2 kcal/min (arm work)
Heart rate	100–105 beats/min (whole body)
	90–95 beats/min (arm work)
Postural stress	Acceptable limit depends on percent maximum voluntary contraction, exertion time, and recovery time.
Perceived stress	Light

Adapted from Garg, A. Manual material handling: The science in *Musculoskeletal Disorders in the Workplace: Principles and Practice,* Nordine, M., Andersson, G., and Pope, M., eds. St. Louis: Mosby, 85–119, 1997. With permission.

Table 13.2   NIOSH Equation

Recommended Weight Limit Computed by Determining:

Horizontal and vertical location of load
Vertical travel distance of load
Frequency and duration of the task
Angular displacement of load
Coupling of load

Table 13.3   NIOSH Equations

Risk of injury increases when:

Heavy objects are lifted
Horizontal location of the hands increases (increased forward reaching)
Vertical location of the hands close to the floor (hands are close to the floor when initiating lifting)
Vertical travel distance of the hands from the beginning of the lift to the endpoint of the lift increases
Object is lifted frequently
Angular displacement of load increases (asymmetric lifting/twisting)
Coupling is poor (poor grip)

Although the NIOSH guidelines are frequently utilized in industry, there is still no universally accepted method of determining a safe lifting capacity for workers. The revised NIOSH equation does have limitations and it has not yet been fully validated.[139]

Despite a lack of validated assessment tools, job design is considered the most effective means of prevention for low back injuries in the workplace.[44, 124] Snook et al. noted in a retrospective study that job design can reduce back injuries associated with manual handling tasks by 33%.[124] Additionally, a worker was three times more likely to injure their back if they were performing tasks that were too difficult for 75% of the population.[125] Snook also found that reducing lumbar flexion (bending) in the early morning at work may reduce the pain and costs associated with chronic low back pain.[127] A prospective epidemiologic study evaluating nursing assistants in a nursing home noted a 50% reduction in the incidence rate for back injuries after a job design program was implemented.[48] The program included mechanical aids and other interventions to reduce the physical demands of the job. The authors also reported that there were no lost or restricted work days due to back injuries after the ergonomics intervention. A population based randomized study of subacute occupational low back pain showed faster return-to-work rates with the addition of occupational interventions which included an ergonomic evaluation.[89]

Ergonomic job design may be the most effective means of preventing occupational low back pain. However, there is still a lack of controlled studies

Table 13.4 Prevention Strategies for Occupational Low Back Pain or Disability

Strategies	Efficacy
Ergonomics	+
Worker Selection	−
Education and Training	−>+
Exercise	+>−
Risk Factor Modification	?
Orthotics	−

+ = Efficacious.
− = Not efficacious.
+>− = Majority of literature support strategy as effective for prevention.
−>+ = Majority of literature does not support strategy as effective for prevention.
? = Efficacy unclear.

evaluating the efficacy of ergonomics for low back pain prevention. Several authors have reported the importance of reducing the physical demands of the job so that they are within the physical capacity of most of the working population.[17, 26, 28, 45, 100, 123, 126] Others argue that it is not clear how beneficial job design is with respect to reducing the incidence of low back injuries.[41, 42] Still others argue that setting limits on lifting will have little impact on the incidence of low back pain although it may have a significant impact on disability by enabling the worker with low back symptoms or dysfunction to remain on the job.[117, 122]

The lack of availability of meaningful ergonomic studies may be due to a number of reasons: 1) generally, high costs of intervention; 2) lack of participation and commitment to ergonomic principles; 3) difficulty in identifying the specific ergonomic changes needed; 4) uncertainty as to what outcome parameters to use; and 5) poor study protocols.[41] While job design may hold the most promise as a prevention strategy for occupational low back pain, debate continues as to whether ergonomic intervention is effective at the primary prevention level or whether ergonomic efforts should focus on secondary and tertiary levels of prevention of low back pain.

13.3.2   Worker Selection

Employers use preemployment screening primarily to attempt to identify those individuals who are at increased risk for low back injuries. Three common methods of worker selection are preemployment strength testing, medical history/physical examination, and radiologic screening.

Preemployment screening has considerable medicolegal ramifications. Preemployment clinical information cannot be used to preclude an individual from working if that worker can physically perform the essential tasks of the job for which he or she is applying.[134] Nonetheless, employers continue to use the worker selection strategies described below in an effort to prevent low back pain.

13.3.2.1   Preemployment Strength Testing

Preemployment strength testing is a controversial screening method still utilized by employers. Several methods of testing strength are utilized including isometric, isokinetic or isoinertial methods. The issue of which is the most appropriate type of test is debated in the literature.[11, 34, 53, 68, 69, 76, 104, 107, 108, 114, 121] Numerous studies have advocated the use of preemployment strength testing as a screening method to reduce low back injuries in the workplace.[25, 27, 68, 69, 114] However, numerous studies have likewise shown that preemployment strength testing is ineffective as a screening tool, whether isometric[8, 104] or isokinetic and isoinertial testing methods are used.[39, 107, 108] Mooney et al.[104] prospectively evaluated shipyard workers and found that preplacement isometric lumbar extensor strength is not a predictor of workplace injury. The authors found that the incidence of back injury claims was highest for the higher physical job demand classifications. There may be a risk associated with preemployment strength testing, therefore, in that it leads to the selection of certain individuals for more physically demanding work based upon the erroneous assumption that their strength will protect them from subsequent back injuries.[90]

13.3.2.2   Medical History/Physical Examination

The most common screening technique used in industry is still the preemployment clinical examination.[13] The primary objective of this examination is to isolate those individuals with previous back disorders. One large prospective study evaluated the effectiveness of the preemployment history and physical examination as a screening method for acute industrial back pain.[13] While the authors reported risk factors for occupational low back pain based on an individual's history, they found that the physical examination findings added no significant predictive value for future low back pain.

An additional prospective study evaluating applicants for light duty work at a telephone company reported similar results.[2] The authors concluded that a preplacement medical evaluation for light duty assignments was not predictive for future work attendance or job performance and was not found to be cost effective.

13.3.2.3   Radiologic Screening

Preplacement radiography to screen out individuals thought to be at greater risk for low back injuries has been a controversial topic. The practice of preplacement screening radiography has fallen out of favor, although some companies still utilize this method to evaluate potential employees. While spondylolisthesis may be a radiographic abnormality seen more often in those with low back pain than in asymptomatic individuals,[51] the majority of the scientific literature reports that screening radiography is not predictive for future low back pain.[16, 51, 52, 79, 116]

There are likely many reasons for the lack of predictive value for radiographs. Plain x-rays tend to correlate poorly with most low back disorders.[16, 79] Symptomatic individuals frequently have normal spine

X-rays while asymptomatic volunteers frequently demonstrate abnormalities on plain X-rays. Also, x-ray findings rarely alter a clinician's treatment plan. The cost of spinal X-rays usually outweighs the potential benefits[116] that are obtained for most low back disorders, particularly in the occupational setting. Furthermore, the etiology of low back pain is often multifactorial in the industrial setting,[14] and in a majority of cases a specific anatomic etiology for low back pain may be elusive even with imaging studies. For these reasons, spinal X-rays are not recommended as a screening tool to prevent low back pain.

13.3.3 Education and Training

Educating and training the worker are primary prevention strategies utilized by industry to prevent low back injuries in the workplace. Education techniques range from simply providing workers with printed material about lifting techniques to the more comprehensive "back schools." The education of supervisors and management is considered an important aspect of secondary and tertiary prevention of low back pain and disability.

13.3.3.1 Lifting Techniques

Jobs that require lifting, especially repetitive and heavy lifting, are associated with an increased risk for low back pain.[45] Several factors have been considered in evaluating lifting techniques, including the compressive forces on the lumbar spine, energy expenditure, ratings of perceived exertion, lifting strength, and productivity. In an effort to lessen the risk for low back injuries, numerous lifting techniques have been described and recommended.[1, 3, 23, 47, 110, 123] Examples include the squat, stoop, and free-style lifting postures. Although a few studies have reported benefits of certain techniques based on biomechanical and physiologic data,[1, 3, 110] there is still no consensus on the safest lifting technique with respect to the prevention of occupational low back pain.[6, 46, 47, 128] Prospective studies that have compared workers trained to use certain lifting techniques to those without such training have reported contradictory results with respect to low back pain prevention in the workplace.[32, 40, 57, 137, 141] Most of the studies noted no significant differences between the trained and untrained groups. Furthermore, some commonly prescribed lifting techniques, such as the squat lifting posture, may actually be detrimental under certain working conditions.[44]

While a specific lifting technique for all lifting tasks cannot be recommended at this time, there are several practical recommendations that can be made. Keeping the lifted object as close as possible to the center of gravity of the body is a biomechanical principle well-supported in the literature[6, 83] (Figure 13.1). Other recommendations include pivoting with the feet instead of twisting with the load, lifting in a smooth and controlled manner, and avoiding overexertion.[44] The use of mechanical aides, such as a hoist, may also prevent some forms of low back pain in the workplace by reducing the load and postural stress.

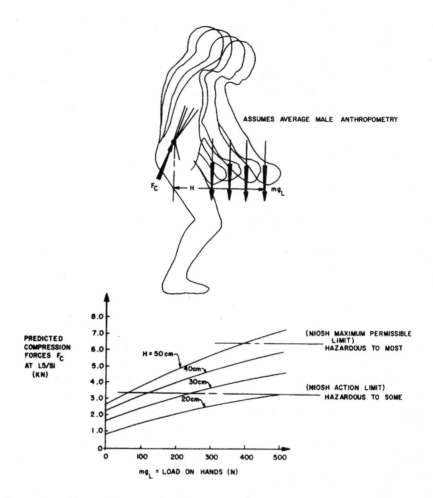

Figure 13.1 The predicted L5/S1 disc compression forces for varying loads in four different positions of the spine. As the lifted load is moved farther from the body (horizontal (H) distance from L5/S1 to the center of grasp increases) the predicted compression forces at L5/S1 increases. From Occupational Biomechanics, Second Edition, Editors Chaffin, D., Andersson, G. John Wiley & Sons, Inc. 1991. Reprinted by permission of John Wiley & Sons, Inc. With permission.

13.3.3.2   Back Schools

Back school programs vary in complexity and format but usually incorporate a group setting. Comprehensive back schools usually consist of one to two day programs, although they may last longer, and most occur on-site at the workplace. These education programs are most frequently utilized at the primary level, but are also incorporated at secondary and tertiary levels. The goals of education programs for workers include establishing a greater knowledge of injury prevention strategies, emphasizing the importance of compliance with treatment programs, and developing an understanding that back pain is usually a benign and self-limited condition. The more comprehensive programs educate individuals about anatomy and physiology, mechanisms of injury, the natural history of disorders, fitness, stress and pain relationships, risk factor modification, proper posture, and body mechanics for material and nonmaterial handling activities.

The efficacy of educational programs for the prevention of low back pain is contradictory in the literature. Physician-directed education about low back pain in symptomatic patients appears to be helpful by increasing patient compliance, reducing health care utilization, and increasing patient satisfaction in the general population.[36, 63, 115] It also may reduce sick leave in the occupational setting.[61] However, the efficacy of structured back schools in the workplace is unproven. Controlled studies report contradictory results with respect to back school and low back pain prevention.[30, 38, 71, 77, 80, 95, 103, 136] A randomized, controlled study evaluated the effectiveness of an education program designed to prevent low back injury in 4,000 postal workers.[31] The education program consisted of a back school followed by three to four reinforcement sessions. The followup period was 5.5 years. The authors reported that the education program "did not reduce the rate of low back injuries, the median cost per injury, the time off of work per injury, or the rate of repeated injury after return to work." Furthermore, a metanalysis regarding back schools noted insufficient evidence to support conclusively the use of back schools.[87] Currently, there is little evidence to support the use of structured educational strategies to prevent low back pain in the workplace.

13.3.3.3 Management Training

Employers, managers, and supervisors may play an important role in the prevention of occupational low back pain. Garg and Moore[47] described potentially effective prevention strategies that can be utilized by management. These include a "positive acceptance" of worker-reported low back pain, a company policy of encouraging workers to report all episodes of low back pain, early intervention and conservative treatment, appropriate follow-up of the worker's treatment and progress, keeping the injured employee at work in some capacity, job analysis, and the enforcement of safety rules. Key barriers to the secondary and tertiary prevention of occupational low back pain include delays in the onset of treatment, reliance upon inappropriate decision makers for returning an employee to work or an inadequate return-to-work plan, limited return-to-work alternatives, inappropriate use of disability determination guidelines, failure to recognize the psychosocial aspects of disability, and a lack of a coordinated effort by the employer, employee and physician.[102]

Clinical trials have underscored the importance of formulating a return-to-work plan during rehabilitation efforts by reporting better return-to-work rates[24] and less subsequent disability.[118] Similar beneficial effects of a return-to-work plan within the chronic pain population have been reported.[94] Hall et al.[56] extended the philosophy of an early return to work for symptomatic patients even further by noting in a prospective study that the probability of a successful return to regular duty work increased with the recommendation of returning to work without restrictions. The probability of failure increased when restrictions were outlined.

The socioeconomic implications of a delayed return to work are well-known. The majority of all costs for occupational low back pain are related to indemnity costs,[140] underscoring the importance of secondary and tertiary prevention and a return-to-work strategy. This, combined with the fact that the probability of an injured worker ever returning to the job decreases as the length of time off work increases,[97] has serious consequences for the system. Certainly it is the physician's role to determine work capacity and an appropriate return-to-work plan. However, industry should be a willing and able partner in this difficult process.

13.3.4   Exercise

Exercise for injury prevention and general well-being has been encouraged by many employers for years. The general health benefits of exercise are well know. Whether exercise can prevent occupational low back pain injury, though, is a more complex question. Exercise programs have focused on the development of strength, flexibility, and endurance. Various types of exercise regimens have been investigated including stretching regimens, calisthenics, strengthening exercises, weight training, aerobics, work simulation/conditioning, and computer-assisted training.

Researchers have reported contradictory results with respect to the effectiveness of exercise for low back pain prevention in the workplace. A few studies have evaluated the efficacy of exercise for the primary prevention of low back pain. One such prospective study[21] evaluated firefighters with no history of low back pain. After four years of observation, the authors concluded that the more physically fit firefighters clearly had lower injury rates. The same authors evaluated back-related medical costs, comparing workers with different degrees of flexibility and back strength. Firefighters with less flexible backs had medical costs seven times higher than their more flexible counterparts; those with weaker backs had a threefold increase in back-related medical costs.[22]

Trunk muscle weakness as a risk factor for low back pain has been studied. Two prospective studies have yielded contradictory results. Mostardi et al.[105] reported that trunk muscle weakness did not correlate with the incidence of low back pain. However, more recently Lee et al.,[81] after a 5-year prospective study, reported that an imbalance of trunk muscle strength involving the lumbar extensor and flexors muscles is one of the risk factors for the incidence of low back pain.

The effectiveness of exercise for secondary and tertiary prevention of low back pain has been evaluated in other studies. Although the reported findings are somewhat contradictory, exercise appears to have a beneficial effect for the prevention of low back pain.[37, 75, 120] Exercising was most beneficial when specifically customized for specific conditions.[120] The greater the intensity of the exercises, the greater the benefit to the individual.[93] Exercise also was noted to be beneficial only as long as it was practiced; discontinuation of the exercise program resulted in no sustainable benefit to the individual.[37]

Furthermore, the benefits of exercise for secondary and tertiary prevention of low back pain have been reported in several controlled studies including those reporting a reduction in symptoms and a statistically significant decrease in missed work days due to low back pain.[38, 55, 67] A randomized comparative multicenter trial evaluated the effects of exercise in patients with low back pain.[88] The 12-month supervised stretching and strengthening program was individualized, with some patients using a training apparatus. The authors reported that the exercise programs led to a significant reduction in absenteeism (75–80%). The benefit from the exercise program persisted during the subsequent unsupervised 12-month follow-up period, even though compliance with the program diminished. However, there are other studies that have reported limited benefits of exercise for low back pain prevention.[8–10, 29, 32, 33]

Other studies have evaluated combined strategies for prevention of low back pain. Bergquist-Ullman and Larsson[12] studied autoworkers with recent back injuries and divided them into three groups: 1) back school with active exercise; 2) active exercise with manual therapy; and 3) passive modalities. There was no significant difference in the recurrences of low back pain nor the number of sick days due to LBP between the groups within 1 year after completing the initial treatment. However, the length of symptom duration was significantly less for the active exercise groups. Another study analyzing the effects of combining prevention strategies on low back pain prevention was reported by Lindstrom et al.[85] The randomized prospective investigation evaluated Swedish automobile workers with an eight-week sick leave due to subacute nonspecific mechanical low back pains.[85] The studied group underwent a graded exercise program, back education, functional capacity measurements, and a worksite evaluation. During the two-year follow-up, the studied group had significantly less sick leave due to low back pain.

In addition, other controlled studies have reported the benefits of combined prevention regimens.[86, 94, 131] Improvements included a reduction of symptoms, a reduction in recurrent low back pain, improved function, and diminished sick leave or an earlier return to work.

Further controlled and randomized studies need to be performed to elucidate the value of exercise for low back pain prevention. Defining which outcome parameters are most important is also necessary because there are a multitude of studies with different assessment methods.[66]

Although the efficacy of exercise for occupational low back pain prevention has been questioned by some investigators, it appears that a higher level of fitness may provide a protective effect against low back injury and does seem to correlate with a more rapid resolution of symptoms and an earlier return to work. Despite the questions that remain concerning the role of exercise and the prevention of occupational low back pain, health care providers and employers should not hesitate to encourage workers to exercise daily due to the many known derived health benefits.

13.3.5   Risk Factor Modification

An individual's anthropomorphic characteristics and personal habits may be associated with the development of low back pain. Several potential risk factors and their association with low back pain have been studied including a person's age, sex, posture, spinal mobility, strength and fitness, weight and tobacco usage.[4] Smoking and obesity are modifiable risk factors that have been of particular interest.

Both smoking[4, 19, 35, 75] and obesity[4, 35, 75] have been linked to low back pain in prospective and cross-sectional studies. However, because it is not clear whether a direct physiologic causal relationship exists, it is unclear whether a modification of these risk factors can lead to prevention of low back pain. Nonetheless, encouraging workers to improve their general health by normalizing their weight and stopping smoking is time well spent.

13.3.6   Lumbar Orthotics

The use of lumbar orthotics for low back injury prevention in the workplace persists despite its controversial status. The theoretical biomechanical advantages of a lumbar corset include an increase in intra-abdominal pressure and subsequent reduction in spinal loading during job tasks, limitation of spinal movement, and an increase in the lifting capacity for individuals. These theoretical benefits, however, are generally not supported by the most recent scientific literature.[44] Most studies have reported that intra-abdominal pressure does not play a significant role in reducing the load on the spine and supporting back and abdominal musculature.[44] Furthermore, lumbar corsets do not have a significant effect on intra-abdominal pressure.[44]

The effect of lumbar corsets on range of motion is contradictory in the literature. Authors have reported that lumbar orthotics reduce the gross range of motion of the lumbar spine.[54, 78, 111] Other authors have reported that lumbar orthotics do not have a stabilizing effect on the intervertebral mobility of the lower lumbar spine and may actually lead to a paradoxical increase in the level of intervertebral motion in certain individuals.[7]

Furthermore, there is limited data on the interaction between lumbar orthotics and lifting capacity. McCoy et al.[96] studied back belts and manual lifting and concluded that back belts increased a worker's perceived maximum acceptable weight lifting compared to the perceived weight lifting without the use of a lumbar orthosis. However, there was insufficient data to predict reliably how a worker's risk of low back injury would be affected by this change in perception. Other authors have reported that lumbar belts do not have a significant effect on lifting capacity.[142] Also, it has been reported that back belts do not reduce lumbar paraspinal muscle fatigue.[92]

One study has evaluated the effects of a lumbar brace on trunk proprioception.[99] Asymptomatic individuals wearing Neoprene lumbar braces were evaluated during flexion of the trunk in the sagittal plane. The authors concluded that lumbar bracing can improve proprioception in asymptomatic individuals. Whether improving trunk proprioception can prevent low back pain and lumbar injury is unknown though.

The usefulness of lumbar orthotics for the prevention of low back pain in the workplace has been evaluated in only a few clinical studies. One such study involved a retrospective review of 1,316 workers who performed lifting activities on a military base.[101] The authors reported that back belts were only minimally effective at preventing injury.[101] Furthermore, the overall cost per injury was substantially higher for workers who had been wearing a back belt compared to those who were not wearing a back belt. The authors concluded that back belt use was not efficacious or cost-effective for low back injury prevention.

In addition, two controlled studies evaluated the use of lumbar orthotics. Walsh and Schwartz[138] published a randomized observer-blinded protocol using grocery warehouse workers. Three groups were evaluated: 1) those completing an education program; 2) those receiving both an education program and a lumbar corset; and 3) a control group. While there was a statistically significant decrease in lost work days for the group that received both education and the lumbar corset, there was no significant difference with respect to the low back injury rate and productivity. It is unclear whether the reduced absenteeism was due to the education program, the lumbar corset or a combination of the two.

Another controlled study evaluating the use of lumbar orthotics by baggage handlers was reported by Reddell.[113] The study groups included: 1) individuals with a lumbar belt; 2) those receiving one hour of training; 3) those receiving both the belt and one hour of training; and 4) a control group. The authors noted no significant difference among the groups with regard to the low back injury rate, or lost or restricted workdays.

While there is limited scientific evidence to support the use of orthotics for low back injury prevention, there are also potential risks for workers wearing lumbar orthotics. Long term use of a lumbar corset may result in physical dependence and a loss of abdominal muscle tone.[54] Other investigators, however, have reported no adverse effects in terms of abdominal muscle strength from wearing lumbar orthoses.[59, 98, 138] An increase in low back injuries and lost work days has also been reported in those individuals who used a lumbar belt and then discontinued its use.[113] Increased worker complaints from the direct effects of the orthosis itself have also been reported.[113, 138] Studies have also reported that lumbar orthoses can adversely effect the cardiovascular system by increasing systolic blood pressure and heart rate.[60, 112] A worker may be at even greater risk when using a lumbar orthosis because the individual may attempt to lift more weight[78] due to the inappropriate perception that an orthosis provides increased security.

In summary, there is no conclusive scientific literature available to support the use of lumbar orthotics in the workplace. Although it is unlikely that there are any severe adverse effects from using a lumbar orthosis in healthy workers, there is no convincing evidence to suggest that the use of lumbar orthotics is an effective prevention strategy.

13.4 Summary

The overwhelming socioeconomic impact and prevalence of occupational low back pain has stimulated the search for effective ways to prevent its occurrence. Among the strategies to prevent occupational low back pain, only job design/redesign and exercise programs appear to have a protective effect (Table 13.4). The majority of the scientific literature supports the use of ergonomics and exercise for prevention of low back pain or disability. However, controlled trials evaluating ergonomic interventions are scarce and the studies pertaining to exercise remain contradictory. Risk factor modification certainly is beneficial from a general health perspective, but the studies are contradictory with respect to its role in the prevention of low back pain. Although certain habits such as smoking are linked with low back pain, the existence of a direct causal relationship is unknown.

Although general education about the benign nature of most low back disorders appear to be helpful, there is no conclusive evidence to support the use of structured education programs or back schools in the workplace, and at this time the cost of the programs is not justified. Furthermore, there is no scientific support for the use of orthotics or worker selection methods based on the available data, and these methods should not be employed in the workplace.

Despite efforts from the medical community and industry, there is little evidence that there has been a substantial impact on the prevalence of low back pain and disability. Perhaps a greater emphasis and job design and exercise can change this trend. Further work is needed in both the occupational and nonoccupational settings to determine effective prevention strategies for low back pain in the future.

13.5 References

1. Adams, M. A. and Hutton, W. C. The effect of posture on the lumbar spine. *J. Bone Joint Surg.* 67-B(4):625–629, 1985.
2. Alexander, R. W., Brennan, J. C., Maida, A. S. et al. The value of preplacement medical examinations for nonhazardous light duty work. *J. Occup. Med.* 19:107–112, 1977.
3. Anderson, C. K., Chaffin, D. B. A biomechanical evaluation of five lifting techniques. *Appl. Ergonomics* 17(1):2–8, 1986.

4. Andersson, G. B. J. The epidemiology of spinal disorders, in *The Adult Spine: Principles and Practice*, Frymoyer, J. W. ed. 93–142, 1997.
5. Andersson, G. B. J. Epidemiologic aspects on low back pain in industry. *Spine* 6:53–60, 1981.
6. Andersson, G. B. J., Ortengren, R., and Nachemson, A. Quantitative studies of back loads in lifting. *Spine* 1(3):178–185, 1976.
7. Axelsson, P. and Johnsson, R. Effect of lumbar orthosis on intervertebral mobility: A roentgen stereophotogrametric analysis. *Spine* 17(6):678–681, 1992.
8. Battie, M. C., Bigos, S. J., Fischer, L. D. et al. Isometric lifting strength as a predictor of industrial back pain reports. *Spine* 14:851–6, 1989.
9. Battie M. C., Bigos, S. J., Fischer, L. D. et al. A prospective study of the role of cardiovascular risk factors and fitness in industrial back pain complaints. *Spine* 14:141–7, 1989.
10. Battie, M. C., Bigos, S. J., Fischer, L. D. et al. The role of spinal flexibility in back pain complaints within industry. *Spine* 15:769–773, 1990.
11. Beimborn, D. S. and Morrissey, M. C. A review of the literature related to trunk muscle performance. *Spine* 13:655–60, 1987.
12. Bergquist-Ullman, M. and Larsson, U. Acute low back pain in industry. *Acta. Orthop. Scand.* 170 (suppl):1–113, 1977.
13. Bigos, S. J., Battie, M. C., Fisher, L. D. et al. A prospective evaluation of pre-employment screening methods for acute industrial back pain. *Spine* 17(8):922–926.
14. Bigos, S. J., Battie, M. C., Spengler, D. M. et al. A longitudinal, prospective study of industrial back injury reporting. *Clin. Orthopaed. Rel. Res.* (279):21–34, 1992.
15. Bigos, S. J., Battie, M. C., Spengler, D. M. et al. A prospective study of industrial work perceptions and psychosocial factors affecting the report of back injury. *Spine* 16:1–6, 1991.
16. Bigos, S. J., Hansson, T., Castillo, R. N., Beecher, P. J., and Wortley, M. D. The value of pre-employment roentgenographs for predicting acute back injury claims and chronic back pain disability. *Clin. Orthop. Rel. Res.* 283:124–9, 1992.
17. Bink, B. The physical working capacity in relation to working time and age. *Ergonomics* 5–25, 1962.
18. Bongers, P. M., deWinter, D. R., Kompier, M. A. J., and Hildebrandt, V. H. Psychosocial factors at work and musculoskeletal disease. *Scan. J. Work Environ. Health* 19:297–312, 1993.
19. Boshuizen, H. C., Verbeek, A. M., Broersen, J. P. J., and Wee, A. N. A. Do smokers get more back pain? *Spine* 18:35–40, 1993.
20. Burton, A. K. Back injury and work loss: Biomechanical and psychosocial influences. *Spine* 22(21):2575–2580, 1997.
21. Cady, L. D., Bischoff, D. P., O'Connell, E. R., Thomas, P. C., and Allan, J. H. Strength and fitness and subsequent back injuries in firefighters. *J. Occup. Med.* 21:269–72, 1979.
22. Cady, L. D., Thomas, P. C., and Karwasky, R. J. Program for increasing health and physical fitness of firefighters. *J. Occup. Med.* 27:110–14, 1985.
23. Calliet, R. *Low Back Pain Syndrome*, 4th ed. Philadelphia: F. A. Davis, 1988.
24. Catchlove, R. and Cohen, K. Effects of a directive return to work approach in the treatment of workman's compensation patients with chronic pain. *Pain* 14:181–191, 1982.

25. Chaffin, D. B. Human strength capability and low back pain. *J. Occup. Med.* 16(4):248–254, 1974.

26. Chaffin, D. B. and Andersson, G. *Occupational Biomechanics.* New York: Wiley, 1991.

27. Chaffin, D. B., Herrin, G. D., and Keyserling, W. M. Preemployment strength testing: An updated position. *J. Occup. Med.* 20:403–408, 1978.

28. Chavalitsakulchai, P. and Shahnavaz, H. Ergonomics method for prevention of the musculoskeletal discomforts among female industrial workers: Physical characteristics and work factors. *J. Human Ergol.* 22:95–113, 1993.

29. Cox, M., Shephard, R. J., and Corey, P. Influence of an employee fitness program upon fitness, productivity, and absenteeism. *Ergonomics* 24:795–806, 1981.

30. Daltroy, L. H., Iversen, M. D., Larson, M. G. et al. Teaching and social support: Effects on knowledge, attitudes, and behaviors to prevent low back injuries in industry. *Health Educ. Q.* 20:43–62, 1993.

31. Daltroy, L. H., Iversen, M. D., Larson, M. G. et al. A controlled trial of an educational program to prevent low back injuries. *N. Engl. J. Med.* 337(5):322–328, 1997.

32. Dehlin, O., Berg, S., Hedenrud, B., Andersson, G. B. J., and Grimby, G. Effect of physical training and ergonomic counseling on the psychological perception of work and on the subjective assessment of low back insufficiency. *Scan. J. Rehabil. Med.* 13:1–9, 1981.

33. Dehlin, O., Berg, S., Hedenrud, B., Andersson, G. B. J., and Grimby, G. Muscle training, psychological perception of work and low back symptoms in nurses' aides. *Scan. J. Rehabil. Med.* 10:201–209, 1978.

34. Delitto, A., Rose, S. J., Crandell, C. E., and Strube, M. J. Reliability of isokinetic measurements of trunk muscle performance. *Spine* 16:800–3, 1991.

35. Deyo, R. A. and Bass, J. E. Lifestyle and low back pain. The influence of smoking and obesity. *Spine* 14:501–6, 1989.

36. Deyo, R. A. and Diehl, A. K. Patient satisfaction with medical care for low back pain. *Spine* 11(1):28–30, 1986.

37. Dillingham, T. R. and DeLateur, B. J. Exercise for low back pain: What really works. *Phys. Med. and Rehabil. State of the Art Rev.* 9:697–708, 1995.

38. Donchin, M., Woolf, O., Kaplan, L., and Floman, Y. Secondary prevention of low back pain: A clinical trial. *Spine* 15:1317–1320, 1990.

39. Dueker, J. A., Ritchie, S. M., Knox, T. J., and Rose, S. J. Isokinetic trunk testing and employment. *JOM* 36(1):42–48, 1994.

40. Feldstein, A., Valanis, B., Vollmer, W., Stevens, N., and Overton, C. The back injury prevention project pilot study: Assessing the effectiveness of back attack: An injury prevention program among nurses, aides, and orderlies. *J. Occup. Med.* 35:114–120, 1993.

41. Frank, J. W., Kerr, M. S., Brooker, A. S. et al. Disability resulting from occupational low back pain. Part I: what do we know about primary prevention? A review of the scientific evidence on prevention before disability begins. *Spine* 21:2908–17, 1996.

42. Frank, J. W., Kerr, M. S., Brooker, A. S. et al. Disability resulting from occupational low back pain. Part II: what do we know about secondary prevention? A review of the scientific evidence on prevention after disability begins. *Spine* 21:2918–29, 1996.

43. Frymoyer, J. W. Cost and control of industrial musculoskeletal injuries, in *Musculoskeletal Disorders in the Workplace Principles and Practice*, Nordin, M., Andersson, G. and Pope, M., eds. Chicago: Mosby, 62–71, 1997.

44. Garg, A. Manual material handling: The science, in *Musculoskeletal Disorders in the Workplace Principles and Practice*, Nordin, M., Andersson, G. and Pope, M., eds. Chicago: Mosby, 1997.

45. Garg, A., Chaffin, D. B., and Herrin, G. D. Predictions of metabolic rates of manual materials handling jobs. *Am. Ind. Hyg. Assoc. J.* 39:661–74, 1978.

46. Garg, A. and Herrin, G. D. Stoop or squat: A biomechanical and metabolic evaluation. *AIIE Transactions*, 11(4):293–302, 1979.

47. Garg, A. and Moore, J. S. Prevention strategies and the low back in industry. *Occup. Med. State of the Art Rev.* 7(4), 1992.

48. Garg, A. and Owen, B. Reducing back stress to nursing personnel: An ergonomic intervention in a nursing home. *Ergonomics* 35:1353–1375, 1992.

49. Gatchel, R. J., Polatin, P. B., and Mayer, T. G. The dominant role of psychosocial risk factors in the development of chronic low back pain disability. *Spine* 20:2702–9, 1995.

50. Genaidy, A. M., Al-Shedi, A., and Shell, R. L. Ergonomic risk assessment: Preliminary guidelines for analysis of repetition, force, and posture. *J. Human Ergol.* 22:45–55, 1993.

51. Gibson, E. S. The value of preplacement screening radiography of the low back. *Occup. Med. State of the Art Rev.* 7(4), 1992.

52. Gibson, E. S., Martin, M. D., and Terry, C. Y. Incidence of low back pain and pre-placement x-ray screening. *JOM* 22:515, 1980.

53. Graves, J. E., Pollack, M. L., Carpenter, D. M. et al. Quantitative assessment of full range of motion isometric lumbar extension strength. *Spine* 15:289–98, 1990.

54. Grew, N. D. and Deane, G. The physical effect of lumbar spinal supports. *Prosthet. Orthop. Int.* 6:79–87, 1982.

55. Gundewall, B., Liljequist, M., and Hansson, T. Primary prevention of back symptoms and absence from work. *Spine* 18:587–594, 1993.

56. Hall, H., McIntosh, G., Melles, T., Holowachuk, B., and Wai, E. Effect of discharge recommendations on outcome. *Spine* 19(18):2033–2037, 1994.

57. Harber, P., Pena, L., Hsu, P. et al. Personal history, training, and worksite as predictors of back pain of nurses. *Amer. J. Ind. Med.* 25:519–526, 1994.

58. Herrin, G. D., Jaraiedi, M., and Anderson, C. K. Prediction of overexertion injuries using biomechanical and psychophysical models. *Am. Ind. Hyg. Assoc. J.* 47:322–30, 1986.

59. Holmstrom, E. and Moritz, U. Effect of lumbar belts on trunk muscle strength and endurance: A follow-up study of construction workers. *J. Spinal Disord.* 5(3):260–266, 1992.

60. Hunter, G. R., McGuirk, J., Mitrano, N., Pearman, P., Thomas, B., and Arrington, R. The effects of a weight training belt on blood pressure during exercise. *J. Appl. Sport Sci. Res.* 3:13–18, 1989.

61. Indahl, A., Velund, L., and Reikeraas, O. Good prognosis for low back pain when left untampered—a randomized clinical trial. *Spine* 20(4):473–477, 1995.

62. Ingelgard, A., Karlsson, H., Nonas, K. and Ortengren, R. Psychosocial and physical work environment factors at three workplaces dealing with materials handling. *Int. J. Ind. Erg.* 17:209–220, 1996.

63. Jones, S. L., Jones, P. K., and Katz, J. Compliance for low back pain patients in the emergency department: A randomized trial. *Spine* 13(5):553–6, 1988.

64. Juul-Kristensen, B., Fallentin, N., and Ekdahl, C. Criteria for classification of posture in repetitive work by observation methods: A review. *Int. J. Ind. Ergonomics.* 19:397–411, 1997.

65. Kaplansky, B. D., Wei, F. Y., and Reecer, M. V. Prevention strategies for occupational low back pain, in *Low Back Pain. Occup. Med.: State of the Art Rev* Malanga, G. A., ed. 13, 1:33–45, 1988.

66. Kara, B. E. and Conrad, K. M. Back injury prevention interventions in the work place. An integrative review. *Am. Assoc. Occup. Health Nurses. J.* 44:189–96, 1996.

67. Kellett, K. M., Kellett, D. A., and Nordholm, L. A. Effects of an exercise program on sick leave due to low back pain. *Phys. Ther.* 4:283–293, 1991.

68. Keyserling, W. M. Strength testing as a method of evaluating ability to perform strenuous work, in *Chronic Low Back Pain,* Stanton-Hicks, M. and Boas, R., eds. New York: Raven Press, 149, 1982.

69. Keyserling, W. M., Herrin, G. D., and Chaffin, D. B. Isometric strength testing as a means of controlling medical incidents on strenuous jobs. *J. Occup. Med.* 22:332–6, 1980.

70. Khalil, T. M., Abdel-Moty, E. M., Rosomoff, R. S., and Rosomoff, H. L. *Ergonomics in back pain.* New York: Van Nostrand Reinhold, 1993.

71. Klaber, Moffett, J. A., Chase, S. M., Portek, I., and Ennis, J. R. A controlled prospective study to evaluate the effectiveness of a back school in the relief of chronic low back pain. *Spine* 11:120–2, 1986.

72. Kumar, S. Isolated planar trunk strength and mobility measurement for the normal and impaired backs: Part I—the devices. *Int. J. Ind. Ergonomics* 17:81–90, 1996.

73. Kumar, S. Trunk strength and mobility measurement for the normal and impaired backs: Part II — protocol, software logic, and sample results. *Int. J. Ind. Ergonomics* 17:91–101, 1996.

74. Kumar, S. Isolated planar trunk strength measurement in normals: Part III—results and database. *Int. J. Ind. Ergonomics* 17:103–111, 1996.

75. Lahad, A., Malter, A. D., Berg, A. O., and Deyo, R. A. The effectiveness of four interventions for the prevention of low back pain. *JAMA* 272(16): 1286–91, 1994.

76. Langrana, N. A., Lee, C. K., Alexander, H., and Mayott, C. W. Quantitative assessment of back strength using isokinetic testing. *Spine* 9:287–90, 1984.

77. Lankhorst, G. J., Van de Stadt, R. J., Vogelaar, T. W. et al. The effect of the swedish back school in chronic idiopathic low back pain: A prospective controlled study. *Scand. Rehabil. Med.* 15:141–5, 1983.

78. Lantz, S. A. and Schultz, A. B. Lumbar spine orthosis wearing. 1. restriction of gross body motions. *Spine* 11:834–837, 1986.

79. LaRocca, H. and Macnab, I. Value of pre-employment radiographic assessment of the lumbar spine. *Ind. Med.* 39(6):253–8, 1970.

80. Leclaire, R., Esdaile, J. M., Suissa, S. et al. Back school in a first episode of compensated acute low back pain. A clinical trial to assess efficacy and prevent relapse. *Arch. Phys. Med. Rehabil.* 77:673–679, 1996.

81. Lee, J., Hoshino, Y., Nakamura, K., Kariya, Y., Saita, K., and Ito, K. Trunk muscle weakness as a risk factor for low back pain—a five-year prospective study. *Spine* (24)54–57, 1999.

82. Lee, K., Waikar, A., and Aghaazadch. Maximum acceptable weight of lift for side and back lifting. *J. Human Ergol.* 19:3–11, 1990.

83. Leskinen, T. P. J., Stalhammar, H. R., and Kuorinka, I. A. A. A dynamic analysis of spinal compression with different lifting techniques. 26(6):595–604, 1983.

84. Liles, D. H. et al. A job severity index for the evaluation and control of lifting injury. *Hum. Factors* 26:683–694, 1984.

85. Lindstrom, I., Ohlund, C., Eek, C. et al. The effect of graded activity on patients with subacute low back pain: A randomized prospective conical study with an operant-conditioning behavioral approach. *Phys. Ther.* 72:279–90, 1992.

86. Linton, S. J., Bradley, L. A., Jensen, I., Spangfort, E., and Sundel, L. The secondary prevention of low back pain: A controlled study with follow-up. *Pain* 36:197–207, 1989.

87. Linton, S. J. and Kamwendo, K. Low back schools: A critical review. *Phys. Ther.* 67(9):1375–83, 1987.

88. Ljunggren, A. E., Weber, H., Kogstad, O. et al. Effect of exercise on sick leave due to low back pain: A randomized, comparative, long-term study. *Spine* 22(14):1610–1617, 1997.

89. Loisel, P., Abenhaim, L., Durand, P. et al. A population-based, randomized clinical trial on back pain management. *Spine* 22(24):2911–2918, 1997.

90. Magnusson, M. Point of view. *Spine* 21(17):2005, 1996.

91. Magora, A. and Tautsein, I. An investigation to the problem of sick-leave in the patient suffering from low back pain. *Indus. Med. Surg.* 38:398–408, 1969.

92. Majkowski, G. R., Jovag, B. W., Taylor, B. T., Taylor, M. S., Allison, S. C., Stetts, D. M., and Clayton, R. L. The effect of back belt use on isometric lifting force and fatigue of the lumbar paraspinal muscles. *Spine* (23)2104–2109, 1998.

93. Manniche, C., Lundberg, E., Christensen, I. et al. Intensive dynamic back exercises for chronic low back pain: A clinical trial. *Pain* 47:53–63, 1991.

94. Mayer, T. G., Gatchel, R. J., Mayer, H. et al. A prospective two-year study of functional restoration in industrial low back injury: An objective assessment procedure. *JAMA* 258(13):1763–1767, 1987.

95. McCauley, M. The effect of body mechanics instruction on work performance among young workers. *Am. J. Occup. Ther.* 44:402–407, 1990.

96. McCoy, M. A., Congleton, J. J., and Johnson, W. C. The role of lifting belts in manual lifting. *Int. J. Ind. Ergon.* 2:259–266, 1988.

97. McGill, C. M. Industrial back problems: Control program. *J. Occup. Med.* 10:174–178, 1968.

98. McGill, C. M., Norman, R. W., and Sharratt, M. T. The effect of an abdominal belt on trunk muscle activity and intra-abdominal pressure during squat lifts. *Ergonomics* 33:147–160, 1990.

99. McNair, P. J. and Heine, P. J. Trunk proprioception: Enhancement through lumbar bracing. *Arch. Phys. Med. Rehabil.* 80:96–98, 1999.

100. Mital, A. Are manual lifting weight limits based on the physiological approach realistic and practical? in *Trends in Ergonomics/Human Factors IV, Part B*, Asfour SS, ed. New York: Elsevier 973, 1987.

101. Mitchell, L. V., Lawler, F. H., Bowen, D. et al. Effectiveness and cost-effectiveness of employer-issued back belts in areas of high risk for back injury. *JOM* 36(1):90–94, 1994.

102. Mitchell, S. and Leclair, S. Building a working alliance with employers: The politics of work disability, in *Physical Medicine and Rehabilitation Clinics of North America*, E. W. Johnson ed. 3(3):647–663, 1992.

103. Moffett, J. A. K. and Chase, S. M., Portek, I. and Ennis, J. R. A controlled, prospective study to evaluate the effectiveness of a back school in the relief of chronic low back pain. *Spine* 11(2):120–122, 1986.

104. Mooney, V., Kenney, K., Leggett, S., and Holmes, B. Relationship of lumbar strength in shipyard workers to workplace injury claims. *Spine* 21(17):2001–2005, 1996.

105. Mostardi, R. A., Noe, D. A., Kovacik, M. W., and Porterfield, J. A. Isokinetic lifting strength and occupational injury: A prospective study. *Spine* 17:189–93, 1992.

106. National Institute for Occupational Safety and Health. *Work Practices Guide for Manual Lifting.* U.S. Department of Health and Human Services. National Technical Information Service. Washington, DC. PB-82, 1981.

107. Newton, M., Thow, M., Somerville, D. et al. Trunk strength testing with iso-machines. Part 2: experimental evaluation of the Cybex II back testing system in normal subjects and patients with chronic low back pain. *Spine* 18(7):812–824.

108. Newton, M. and Waddell, G. Trunk strength testing with iso-machines. Part 1: review of a decade of scientific evidence. *Spine* 18(7):801–811.

109. Papageorgiou, A. C., MacFarlane, G. J., Thomas, E. et al. Psychosocial factors in the workplace—Do they predict new episodes of low back pain? *Spine* 22:1137–1142, 1997.

110. Parke, K. S. and Chaffin, D. B. A biomechanical evaluation of two methods of manual load lifting. *AIIE Transactions* 6(2):105–113, 1974.

111. Perry, J. The use of external support in the treatment of low back pain. *J. Bone Joint Surg. Am.* 52A(7):1440–1442, 1970.

112. Rafacz, W. and McGill, S. M. Wearing an abdominal belt increases diastolic blood pressure. *JOEM* 38(9):925–927, 1989.

113. Reddell, C. R. Congleton, J. J., Hunchingston, R. D., and Montgomery, J. F. An evaluation of a weightlifting belt and back injury prevention training class for airline baggage handlers. *Appl. Ergon.* 23:319–329, 1992.

114. Reimer, D. S., Halbrook, B. D., Dreyfuss, P. H., and Tibiletti, C. A novel approach to preemployment worker fitness evaluations in a material-handling industry. *Spine* 19:2026–32, 1994.

115. Roland, M. and Dixon, M. Randomized controlled trial of an educational booklet for patients presenting with back pain in general practice. *J. R. Coll. Gen. Pract.* 39(323):244–6, 1989. Spinal injuries—a three-year follow-up study. *Spine* 17(9):1043–1047, 1992.

116. Rowe, M. L. Are routine spine films on workers in industry cost- or risk-benefit effective? *J. Occup. Med.* 24(1):41–43, 1992.

117. Rowe, M. L. Low back disability in industry: Updated position. *J. Occup. Med.* 13(10):476–478, 1971.

118. Sanderson, P. L., Todd, B. D., Holt, G. R., and Getty, C. J. M. Compensation, work status, and disability in low back pain patients. *Spine* 20(5):554–556, 1995.

119. Scheer, S. J. and Mital, A. Ergonomics. *Arch. Phys. Med. Rehabil.* (supp):78:36–45, 1997.

120. Scheer, S. J., Radack, K. L., and O'Brien, D. R., Jr. Randomized controlled trials in industrial low back pain relating to return to work. Part 1, acute interventions. *Arch. Phys. Med. Rehabil.* 76:966–73, 1995.

121. Smith, S. S., Mayer, T. G., Gatchel, R. J., and Becker, T. J. Quantification of lumbar function. Part 1. isometric and multispeed isokinetic trunk strength measures in sagittal and axial planes in normal subjects. *Spine* 10:757–64, 1985.
122. Snook, S. H. Psychophysical considerations in permissible loads. *Ergonomics* 28:327–330, 1985.
123. Snook, S. H. The design of manual handling tasks. *Ergonomics* 21:963–85, 1978.
124. Snook, S. H., Campanelli, R. A., and Hart, J. W. A study of three preventative approaches to low back injury. *J. Occup. Med.* 20:478–81, 1978.
125. Snook, S. H., Irvine, C. H., and Bass, S. F. Maximum weights and work loads acceptable to male industrial workers; A study of lifting, lowering, pushing, pulling, carrying, and walking tasks 579–86, 1970.
126. Snook, S. H. and Ciriello, V. M. Maximum weights and work loads acceptable to female workers. *J. Occup. Med.* 16:527–34, 1974.
127. Snook, S. H., Webster, B. S., McGorry, R. W., Fogleman, M. T., and McCann, K. B. The reduction of chronic nonspecific low back pain through the control of early morning lumbar flexion—a randomized controlled trial. *Spine* 23:2601–2607, 1998.
128. Songcharoen, P., Chotigavanich, C., and Thanapipatsiri, S. Lumbar paraspinal compartment pressure in back muscle exercise. *J. Spinal Disorders* 7(1):49–53, 1994.
129. Straker, L. M. Work-associated back problems: Measurement problems. *J. Soc. Occup. Med.* 41:41–44, 1991.
130. Straker, L. M., Stevenson, M. G., and Twomey, L. T. A comparison of risk assessment of single and combination manual handling tasks. 1. Maximum acceptable weight measures. *Ergonomics* 39:128–40, 1996.
131. Stankovic, R. and Johnell, O. Conservative treatment of acute low back pain. A prospective randomized trial: McKenzie method of treatment versus patient education in "mini back school" *Spine* 15:120–23, 1990.
132. Stobbe, T. J. Occupational ergonomics and injury prevention. *Occup. Med.: State of the Art Rev.* 11(3):531–543, 1996.
133. Symonds, T. L., Burton, A. K., Tillotson, K. M., and Main, C. J. Do attitudes and beliefs influence work loss due to low back trouble? *Occup. Med.* 46:25–32, 1996.
134. The Americans With Disabilities Act of 1990. Pub. L. No. 101–336, 104 Stat 327.
135. U.S. Department of Labor, Bureau of Labor Statistics, April 1996. Survey of Occupational Injuries and Illnesses, 1994.
136. Versloot, J. M., Rozeman, A., van Son, A. M., and van Akkerveeken, P. F. The cost-effectiveness of a back school program in industry: A longitudinal controlled field study. *Spine* 17(1):22–27, 1992.
137. Videman, T., Rauhala, H., Lindstrom, K. et al. Patient-handling skill, back injuries, and back pain—an intervention study in nursing. *Spine* 14(2):148–156, 1989.
138. Walsh, N. E. and Schwartz, R. K. The influence of prophylactic orthoses on abdominal strength and low back injury in the workplace. *Am. J. Phys. Med. Rehabil.* 69:245–250, 1990.
139. Waters, T. R., Putz-Anderson, V., Garg, A., and Fine, L. J. Revised NIOSH equation for the design and evaluation of manual lifting tasks. *Ergonomics* 36:749–76, 1993.

140. Webster, B. S. and Snook, S. H. The cost of 1989 workers' compensation low back pain claims. *Spine,* 19(10):1111–1116, 1993.
141. Wood, D. J. Design and evaluation of a back injury prevention program within a geriatric hospital. *Spine* 12:77–82, 1987.
142. Woodhouse, M. L., Heinen, J., Shall, L. et al. Selected isokinetic lifting parameters of adult male athletes utilizing lumbar/sacral supports. *J. Orthop. Sports. Phys. Ther.* 11(10):467–473, 1990.

Index

Index